CLINICAL
OCULAR
PHOTOGRAPHY

CLINICAL OCULAR PHOTOGRAPHY

Denise Cunningham, COA, CRA, RBP, MEd

Instructor, Department of Ophthalmology
Georgetown University School of Medicine
Director of Ocular Photography and Special Studies
Georgetown University Center for Sight
Washington, DC

▌▌▌ The Basic Bookshelf for Eyecare Professionals

Series Editors: Janice K. Ledford • Ken Daniels • Robert Campbell

SLACK Incorporated, 6900 Grove Road, Thorofare, NJ 08086

Publisher: John H. Bond
Editorial Director: Amy E. Drummond
Creative Director: Linda Baker
Assistant Editor: Elisabeth DeBoer

Cunningham, Denise
    Clinical ocular photography/ by Denise Cunningham.
    p. cm.
    Includes bibliographical references and index.
    ISBN 1-55642-377-2 (alk.paper)
    1. Ophthalmic photography.   I. Title.
    [DNLM: 1. Eye Diseases -- diagonosis. 2. Diagnostic Techniques,
Ophthalmological. 3. Photography -- methods.   WW 141 C973c 1998]
RE79.P54C86 1998
617.7'15 -- dc21
DNLM/DLC
for Library of Congress   98-13365
                                    CIP

Printed in the United States of America
Published by: SLACK Incorporated
               6900 Grove Road
               Thorofare, NJ 08086-9447 USA
               Telephone: 609-848-1000
               Fax: 609-853-5991

Last digit is print number: 10 9 8 7 6 5 4 3 2 1

Dedication

For Ellen, Lily, Evelyn, and Betty—my partner, my daughter, my mother, and my friend.

Contents

Acknowledgments

Having worked as a professional eye photographer for almost 20 years, I am indebted to the many people who have contributed to my knowledge about cameras and eyes. Professors Gus Kayafas and Nicholas Nixon, at the Massachusetts College of Art, were both wonderful examples of working professionals who could inspire through their teaching, as well as their pictures.

As all of my work in ophthalmology has taken place in three different academic medical centers, I have many sets of ophthalmic medical personnel, nurses, medical students, residents, fellows, and attending physicians to thank for teaching me ophthalmology. Although it's been many years since I worked at the Massachusetts Eye and Ear Infirmary, I still have fond memories of fixing Dr. Daniel J. Townsend's bicycle in the emergency room and am forever indebted to Dr. Carmen A. Puliafito for writing a stellar letter of recommendation that got me my great job at Penn State. Jennifer Hamlin taught me well and Chris Gomes made me laugh. Dr. Evangelos S. Gragoudas was a delight to work for.

While at Penn State, Dr. Barton L. Hodes showed tremendous respect for me and my profession by paying me well. Dr. Joseph W. Sassani dispelled my belief that all subspecialists were shortsighted when he diagnosed sleep apnea and a broken neck on two of his glaucoma patients. Working with Dr. Carl A. Frankel and his pediatric patients helped me to become a faster and more agile photographer. If I could photograph "nine positions of gaze" on a two-year-old, then I could photograph anything.

When George W. Blankenship arrived in Hershey to head Penn State's new Department of Ophthalmology, I knew that I was very fortunate both to be part of his team and to witness a gifted surgeon and charismatic leader at work. Dr. Stuart H. Goldberg, a wonderful father, caring husband, and fine man, is a perfect example of what I look for in a doctor. In particular, Dr. George O.D. Rosenwasser stands out in my heart, not only for his significance as my first mentor of cornea and external disease, but because of our longstanding friendship.

All twenty-seven ophthalmologists-in-training with whom I worked at Penn State were special to me, but no one could compare with Dr. Yaron S. Rabinowitz when it came to panache. Dr. Denise M. Visco is an excellent surgeon, a kind and caring physician, and a wonderful friend. I don't remember whether it is his intelligence, his sense of humor, or his equally bright and witty partner, Susanne Scott, that makes Dr. David G. Scott so unforgettable. The surgical scar on my right shoulder reminds me of the unique bond I have with Dr. Raymond DeMaio. My rotator cuff was never the same after his "chiropractic adjustment." (It's a good thing he went into ophthalmology.)

Once-a-week trips to Penn State's VAMC affiliate in Lebanon, Pa, were a welcome departure from my daily routine at Hershey. The clinic's optometry chief, James M. Aylward, OD, FAAO, saw to it that my clinic was well organized and smoothly run while treating me like a visiting "professor."

Marge Michalski, RN, Mary Frawley, COA, and Jean Walker, COA, made it easy to go to work everyday. Marge rarely missed a vein during fluorescein angiography, Mary rarely missed an opportunity to be kind, and Jean rarely missed an interesting discussion.

On the administrative side of things, Marcia Krick and Judy Bowman were always there for me. With his superb managerial skills, Gregory M. Bracale helped shape the department into a first-class operation and occasionally "waxed on philosophically." Judy Ladda just wanted me to be happy.

When Maureen Hargaden, VMD, ACLAM, a doctor of veterinary medicine, and I worked together for a few months on her research with a group of monkeys, I didn't know that we were also working on a friendship.

Ironically, Mr. Daniel T. O'Donnell also worked at Penn State Medical Center during my time there but our professional paths rarely crossed. He contributed greatly to this book, however, with his undying friendship and fabulously prepared gourmet meals.

Since moving to Washington, DC, I've had the pleasure of working with some of the "best and brightest" in ophthalmology. In particular, the quality of the ophthalmic medical personnel at the Center for Sight is outstanding. Phyllis L. Fineburg, COMT, director of Georgetown University's OMP training program, and so many of her students from the classes of 1996-1998 made this book possible by giving me the freedom to use them as models and the slack to not be as attentive to their needs as I should have been whenever I had a book deadline to meet.

Elizabeth A. Burt, COT, is one of the smartest people I know. Merely professional acquaintances before I arrived at Georgetown, we are now very close friends. I am forever indebted to her for both typing and proofreading the many drafts of this book. Because she is a wonderful writer herself, Elizabeth's criticism of my work was most welcome and extremely helpful. Without her aid, this book would still be just another work in progress.

Although Angelina A. Goldman, COT, and I have worked together since I arrived in Washington, our relationship transcends that which is ocular. She's interesting and interested, and her support as my friend has been consistent and constant.

Despite his being officially "retired," Charles Douglas, COMT, has often come to my rescue by covering for me when I needed some concentrated time to work on this book. My only regret about having him work in my place is that I don't get to work alongside him during that time.

Someone that I do have the pleasure of working with on a daily basis is Howard P. Cupples, professor and chair of the Department of Ophthalmology at Georgetown University. Dr. Cupples provided me with precious time to write the words and costly supplies to print the pictures that illustrate this book. His most valuable contribution has been the paternal support that he has given to this tremendous effort.

It is my own father, Francis X. Cunningham, who deserves the biggest share of my thanks. By encouraging me to combine my avocation with an education, he gave me the key to professional happiness.

About the Author

Denise Cunningham is the third of eight children born to Francis X. and Evelyn T. Cunningham. She grew up in Revere, Mass, just north of Boston, and was a student at the Immaculate Conception School for 12 years. In junior high, while enrolled in a drawing and painting class at a local YMCA, she became a serious student of the arts. Her proudest achievement from those early days was an oil portrait of her idol, the legendary rock star, Janis Joplin.

As a high school student, she'd always been fascinated with science but chose instead to concentrate on her artistic interests. As a sophomore, she got her first camera, a Kodak Instamatic, as a birthday gift and became obsessed with chronicling the adventures of her friends and family.

Her second camera, a Fujica ST-701, was given to her by her father as a reward for finishing her freshman year at the Massachusetts College of Art. Although her major was painting, she wanted to learn how to use her camera and registered for an introductory course in photography the following semester. Being seduced by the photographic process, she quickly abandoned her paint brushes and picked up her 35-mm SLR instead, for good. Taking pictures became her passion, as well as her major, and she graduated with a bachelor of fine arts degree in photography.

Having an undergraduate degree in the field didn't translate into a photography job, so she continued to toil as a customer service representative in the catalog division of a large retail merchandiser, a job she held throughout college. One day, while walking home from work, she spotted a dead cat on the road and started taking pictures. After making a few exposures, the light bulb went off in her head, and she knew that she would use her camera to make a living photographing biological subjects—dead or alive.

In the fall of 1978 she enrolled in the School of Medical Photography at Beth Israel Hospital in Boston. As an extern, she gained specialty training in pathology at Massachusetts General Hospital and Harvard Medical School and in ophthalmology at Tuft's New England Medical Center. After completing the one-year program, she was immediately hired to work at the Massachusetts Eye and Ear Infirmary, where she performed fundus photography and fluorescein angiography. After a year of working in the field, she entered the certification program of the Ophthalmic Photographers' Society and succeeded in passing both a written and practical examination to become a certified retinal angiographer (CRA).

Armed with an education in photography, training in medical photography, and experience and certification in ophthalmic photography, Denise left Boston for Hershey, Penn, to head the photography section of the then Division of Ophthalmology at the Pennsylvania State University College of Medicine. While at Penn State, she worked on a master's degree in training and development from the Graduate School of Education and became a certified ophthalmic assistant (COA), a certified ophthalmic photographer and retinal angiographer (COPRA), and a registered biological photographer (RBP). Twelve years later, longing for the city, she left central Pennsylvania and moved to Washington, DC to be the director of ocular photography at Georgetown University's Center for Sight.

In December of 1997, Denise graduated from Pennsylvania State University with a master's degree in education (MEd). She continues to study and teach in the ophthalmic field but is also exploring alternatives to western medicine. As a student at the Potomac Massage Training Institute (PMTI) in Washington, DC, she has found that working as a massage therapist is an excellent complement to her work as a medical photographer. When not in school or at work (or writing a book), Denise spends her time with her loving partner and their wonderful daughter at home in Takoma Park, Md.

Foreword

Photography is a very important component of ophthalmology. Many successful research projects in ophthalmology have relied on photographic documentation to determine the effectiveness of new treatments and to obtain new knowledge about eye diseases and their effects on vision. The ability to document anatomical findings with photographs greatly enhances the quality of care patients receive, for, without a picture, demonstrating the change in size or appearance of ocular abnormality would be more complicated and less accurate. If photographs were not obtained to map out problem areas and guide treatment and follow-up care, a surgical procedure or medical remedy for a variety of sight-threatening conditions would be much less successful.

In addition to their value to ocular scientists and clinicians, photographs also provide students and health care workers with visual examples of the human eye in health and disease. Those who wish to familiarize themselves with some of the basic techniques of film-based imaging of the eye should find this manual, *Clinical Ocular Photography*, to be an excellent introduction. Even those who are using more sophisticated digital equipment should profit from the book's back-to-basics approach. After all, a retina is a retina is a retina, whether its image is recorded with silver or silicon.

It was my great pleasure to be an associate of Ms. Cunningham's at the Penn State's College of Medicine during her 12-year tenure there. Her extensive experience in all aspects of ophthalmic photography, natural and learned skills, and interest in teaching and clinical research, make her well qualified for writing this book, which is readily apparent in its pages. I believe that Denise has been successful by combining a knowledge and understanding of the importance of her work with superb technical skills and a genuine concern for the comfort of her subject—the patient.

George W. Blankenship, MD
Senior Vice President of Clinical Operations
Penn State Geisinger Health System
Department of Ophthalmology
Professor and Chair
Penn State College of Medicine
Hershey, Pa
August 5, 1997

Introduction

I'd never thought about writing a book on ophthalmic photography until Jan Ledford, the editor of this Basic Bookshelf series, approached me about the task in the winter of 1995. After accepting her offer, my ego spent the first few months basking in the glory of being an author, but my hand never picked up a pen. Then, when I finally sat down to do some serious writing, it hit me—I was a visual artist, not a writer. It was no accident that I was taking pictures for a living rather than writing reports since, for me, putting ideas onto a piece of paper that did not have to be handled under safelight illumination was frightening.

Well, over a year and many drafts later, the scary part is finally over for me—the book is finished. My hope is that it will serve to reduce any fear or anxiety that you may have related to learning the craft of ocular photography.

This book was written in a peculiar way. I shot and printed the pictures first and then wrote the words to match these illustrations. As I said, I'm no writer. If the written words are hard to sift through, just look at the pictures. After all, every picture tells a story...

Denise Cunningham, COA, CRA, RBP, MEd

The Study Icons

The Basic Bookshelf for Eyecare Professionals is quality educational material designed for professionals in all branches of eyecare. Because so many of you want to expand your careers, we have made a special effort to include information needed for certification exams. When these study icons appear in the margin of a Series book, it is your cue that the material next to the icon (which may be a paragraph or an entire section) is listed as a criteria item for a certification examination. Please use this key to identify the appropriate icon:

OptA   optometric assistant

OptT   optometric technician

OphA   ophthalmic assistant

OphT   ophthalmic technician

OphMT   ophthalmic medical technologist

LV   low vision subspecialty

Srg   ophthalmic surgical assisting subspecialty

CL   contact lens registry

Optn   opticianry

RA   retinal angiographer

Chapter 1

Scientific Photography

- Standardize your photographic technique to ensure reproducibility.

- Use metric measurements for precision.

- Magnification is how large or small an object is on film.

- Patient management is crucial in clinical photography.

- Patients are people, not diseases.

A Scientific Photograph or a Snapshot?

With the exception of fluorescein angiograms, most photographs taken in a medical setting have little or no diagnostic significance but do have documentary value and are important to both the physician managing a medical condition and the individual patient receiving care. The benefits of obtaining medical photographs are not just limited to a specific doctor or patient. Illustrations are essential to medical educators involved in teaching and research and are invaluable aids for doctors, nurses, and other health care workers who need to recognize the appearance of the many diseases and disorders that affect their patient population. Therefore, we all profit when photographs of the human body, in health and disease, are obtained.

As a parent reaching for a camera to record your baby's first step, you may pick up the exact same make and model of camera selected by the medical photographer to document a patient's foot deformity. The difference between the two photographs lies primarily in the intention of the photographer and the intended use of the image obtained, not in the equipment selected. While a mother's snapshot of her child may fulfill her desire to preserve a special moment and earn itself a place in the family album, it probably won't be viewed by anyone outside the child's intimate circle of family and friends. The medical photograph of a foot, on the other hand, may be seen by literally thousands of people. Although initially taken to accompany a progress note in the patient's chart, the image of the anomaly may appear in an anatomy lecture for medical students, an orthopaedic textbook on locomotion and, if surgery is performed, may later be used as one half of a "before-and-after" series. Because of this, it is especially important for photographers working in the medical field to standardize with the goal of producing a scientific photograph rather than a snapshot (Figure 1-1).

Standardization

Checking visual acuity is an important component of every eye examination and has become standardized for repeatable results. The routine is universal. The patient faces an illuminated test chart at a distance of 6 m (20 ft) and reads down the chart as far as possible. Each eye is checked separately, and the smallest line that can be read is recorded. When photography is included as part of an ocular examination, the conditions under which it is performed should also be standardized using reproducible photographic techniques. Subject positioning, background, angle of view, and magnification must be considered and controlled when photographing a medical subject. Selecting the appropriate camera and choosing a suitable film is also important if your photograph is to serve as an accurate representation of your subject. In short, only the patient or pathology is permitted to vary from one photograph to the next.

What to include in an ocular photograph is best determined by the physician requesting the picture. Perhaps all of Dr. Smith's patients with ptosis will have external eye photographs taken of "both eyes together" in primary position, upgaze, and downgaze. Maybe all glaucoma suspects seen in his or her practice will have "high magnification" photos taken of the optic nerve, and all patients diagnosed with retinal vascular occlusions will have "wide angle" angiography performed, if indicated. It doesn't matter which views the doctor requires to document a specific disease or disorder; what matters is that the photographer is able to replicate these views from visit to visit. Developing standard procedures based on the expectations of the physician, the expertise of the photographer, and the available equipment is recommended to insure reproducibility.

With today's automated camera equipment, you can move buttons and controls without ever

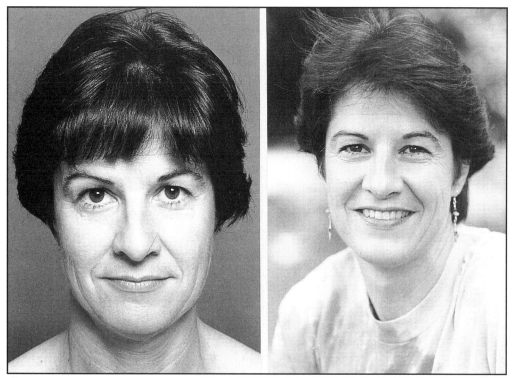

Figure 1-1. Two full face photographs taken of the same subject, at the same distance, using the same camera (Nikon F3) and lens (105mm). Left: A scientific photograph. Right: A snapshot.

knowing what the numbers on these knobs mean and still obtain fairly good results. If your wish is to become proficient in the craft of photography and a competent eye photographer, however, it is important to know what these numbers represent. Don't worry, you do not need a degree in mathematics to avail yourself of the information etched on your camera equipment (Figure 1-2), for no computations or calculations are needed. In most cases, a quick review of the owner's manual is all you'll need to learn which group of numbers are shutter speeds, aperture stops, magnification ratios, etc. If you are more confused after consulting the owner's manual and wonder just how long a millimeter is or what the "X" means in 40X, then you may need to review two important areas in scientific photography: measurement and magnification.

Measurement

The Metric System

When dealing with length in the United States, most people use an adaptation of the British system of measurement, which utilizes the familiar inch, foot, yard, and mile designation. Scientists throughout the world, however, use the metric system of measurement, with the meter (about 39 in) as its basic unit. All measurements in the metric system are fractions or multiples of a meter with units of the same class related to one another by 10 (Table 1-1). This makes computations, comparisons, and conversion from one metric unit to another relatively easy and most precise.

Ophthalmologists make use of metric measurements every time they check intraocular pressure or record the size of a lesion. Even the standard measure of lens power for glasses, the

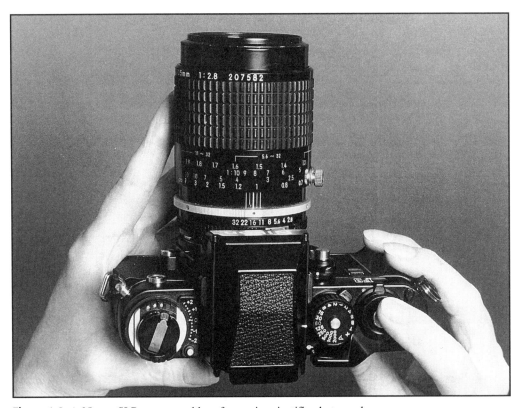

Figure 1-2. A 35-mm SLR camera and lens for use in scientific photography.

diopter, is nothing more than the reciprocal of the focal length of a lens in millimeters. Photographers also utilize the metric system and even include a metric unit of length, the millimeter, in the name of the popular 35-mm camera. Lenses and films are generally described and categorized by their size in millimeters. A millimeter is 1000th of a meter. This can be written as a fraction (1/1000 m), a decimal (00.001 m) or in scientific notation (1×10^{-3} m).

 Scientific Notation

Very large or very small numbers are easily handled using the metric system and scientific notation. A number in scientific notation is expressed as a base number times 10 raised to some power called an exponent. When you "raise a number to a power," you multiply it by itself the number of times the exponent indicates. For example, the number "1000" can be represented mathematically as "1 X 10 X 10 X 10," or written as "1×10^{3}" in scientific notation since both equal 1000. The positive exponent ^{3} tells you that the decimal point must be moved three places to the right of the number one when 1000 is written out as 1000.00. Numbers less than one are represented in scientific notation by means of a negative exponent. This explains why the millimeter, "1000th of a meter," is written as 1×10^{-3} m. The $^{-3}$ tells you that the decimal point is located exactly three places to the left when a millimeter is written in its decimal form as 00.001 m.

Magnification

Photographs taken with the fundus camera, photo slit lamp, and specular microscope almost

Table 1-1

METRIC MEASUREMENTS OF LENGTH

Unit Name	Symbol	Number	Scientific Notation	Fraction	Meaning
kilometer	km	1,000 m	1×10^3 m	1,000/1 m	one thousand meters
hectometer	hm	100 m	1×10^2 m	100/1 m	one hundred meters
decameter	dam	10 m	1×10^1 m	10/1 m	ten meters
meter	m	1 m	1×10^0 m	1/1 m	one meter
decimeter	dm	0.1 m	1×10^{-1} m	1/10 m	one tenth of a meter
centimeter	cm	0.01 m	1×10^{-2} m	1/100 m	one hundredth of a meter
millimeter	mm	0.001 m	1×10^{-3} m	1/1,000 m	one thousandth of a meter
micrometer	μm	0.000001 m	1×10^{-6} m	1/1,000,000 m	one millionth of a meter
nanometer	nm	0.000000001 m	1×10^{-9} m	1/1,000,000,000 m	one billionth of a meter

always depict the subject (the eye) larger than life. On the negative or color slide, the image of the subject is bigger than its actual size in the real world. We call this a magnified image. External eye photographs usually represent the subject smaller than life size. For example, if a photograph is taken to include the patient's head and shoulders, the image on a frame of 35-mm film will be less than the actual size of the subject's head. Interestingly enough, in photography, this reduction in image size is still called magnification. Magnification indicates how much larger or smaller a subject is recorded on the film.

Magnification (M) is the ratio comparing the size of the image (I) of a subject on film to the actual size of the subject (S). For example, if a head measures 24 mm on film but is actually 240 mm in real life, the ratio is 24:240 or, when reduced, 1:10. On some cameras, a reproduction ratio scale (Figure 1-3) is provided so that the lens can be set to an exact magnification ratio. When this scale is used, focusing is achieved by setting the focusing ring to the appropriate reproduction ratio marked on the lens barrel and having the photographer move in towards or back away from the subject until the image is sharp.

Another way to calculate magnification does involve some math. Using the formula $I \div S = M$, divide the image of the head size in the above example (24 mm) by the subject size (240 mm). Your answer will be a fraction, 1/10. Photographic and ophthalmic sources will abbreviate this as 1/10X, with the letter "X" serving as a substitute for the words "times life size." Biomedical photography purists prefer that the letter "X" precede the number when referring to total magnification and would express it as X1/10 instead.[1-2] However it is written, all would describe the magnification in the same words, "one tenth times life size."

If the magnification ratio is 1:1, the image on the film is life size, or the exact same size on the film as in real life. With the exception of external eye photographs, most ophthalmic pictures represent the eye larger than life. When you look through a specialized eye camera, the patient's eye will appear larger to you than it will to the film inside the camera. What you see is called visual, rather than photographic, magnification. Visual magnification is the product of the power of the ocular (eyepiece) multiplied by the power of the objective (lens) in use. Using this equation, a slit lamp with a 12.5X ocular, when used in combination with a 3.2X objective, will afford a 40X view of the subject. In other words, when looking through the microscope, things will appear "40 times life size." This is a "virtual" image, which is visible only in the brain of the observer and cannot be photographed.

A "real" image of the subject is one that exists in space and can be captured photographically. When calculating the magnification of such an image, the projection distance of the camera in use plays a role in image size and must be factored into the formula.[3] Because of this, photographic magnification and visual magnification are not always the same. In the case of the slit lamp, the photographic magnification was much less than what was seen through the eyepiece of the microscope. The subject that appeared 40 times life size through the ocular measured a little less than five times life size (4.8X) on film.

The photographic magnifications obtained with most slit lamp cameras range from approximately 1X to 5X. A conventional 30° fundus camera, on the other hand, is limited to a set magnification of 2.5X when used as is, but an extender placed in front of its 35-mm camera back can double its power to magnify (Figure 1-4). Variable angle fundus cameras offer the user a menu of magnifications from which to choose by the addition of internal accessory lenses. These lenses increase the retinal image size on film from 1.2X to 5X by turning a dial (Figure 1-5). One contact wide field specular microscope, which enlarges the corneal endothelium to an incredible 160X through the eyepiece, depicts this same cell layer at around 40X magnification on a 35-mm

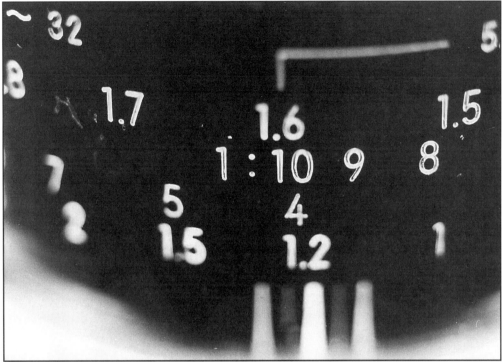

Figure 1-3. This close-up view of the camera lens from Figure 1-2 is centered on the reproduction ratio scale which is set for 1:10.

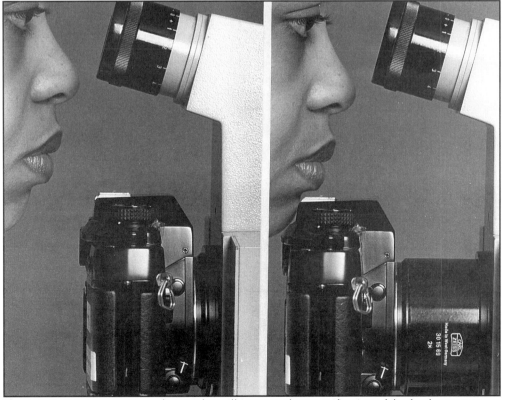

Figure 1-4. Using an accessory lens (right) will increase the magnification of the fundus camera.

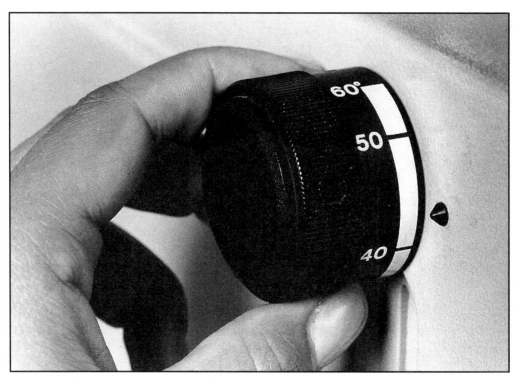

Figure 1-5. Dialing in the desired magnification on a variable angle fundus camera.

film frame. Because "what you see" through the ocular is not "what you get" on film, the owner's manual of the specific make and model of camera being used should be consulted when exact magnifications must be known.

The hand-held positive lenses used in patient examinations are generally referred to by their dioptric designation while camera lenses are customarily described by their focal length in millimeters. Magnifying lenses are labeled by how many times they enlarge their subject. Despite the variation in nomenclature, when using a simple single-element lens, all of these lens types can be converted to and classified by their dioptric power, focal length in millimeters, and their power to magnify (Table 1-2).[4] Surprisingly, a 20 D lens used for indirect ophthalmoscopy has the exact same focal length as a 50-mm camera lens, and the same power as the 5X magnifier used to look at negatives (Figure 1-6). Although they are categorized quite differently and serve dissimilar purposes, these three lenses are essentially the same.

OptT

The Use of Photography in Medicine

Since its inception, photography has been embraced by the medical community. Composite photographs of student doctors, interns, and residents grace the walls of hospitals and medical schools. While they help in identifying the wearers of the white coats, these pictures also provide their subjects with a personal keepsake of their medical training. Photographs depicting practitioners engaged in the science and art of medicine now illustrate newsletters, annual reports, and glossy informational brochures to communicate positive public relations images of the medical community. Despite the popularity and usefulness of these non-clinical images, pictures of patients are still the most valued of medical images for their undisputed importance in the care of patients,

Table 1 - 2

THE SIMPLE LENS

Dioptric Power (D)	=	Focal Length (mm)	=	Magnification (X)
+1		1,000		.25
+2		500		.50
+3		333.33		.75
+4		250		1
+5		200		1.25
+6		166.66		1.50
+7		142.86		1.75
+8		125		2
+9		111.11		2.25
+10		100		2.50
+20		50		5
+28		35.71		7
+60		16.66		15
+78		12.82		19.50
+90		11.11		22.50

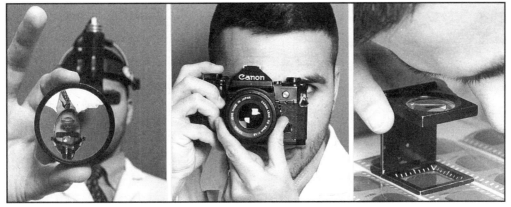

Figure 1-6. A 20 D, 50 mm, and 5x lens in use. Although essentially the same, each lens serves very different needs.

education of health care providers, and furtherance of clinical research.

It has become rather commonplace for patients to be photographed during a visit to the doctor. In fact, "being looked at by doctor, camera, or diagnostic machine is a deeply ingrained visual expectation of the office medical encounter."[5] Like their colleagues in other medical specialties, eye doctors have always been interested in using a camera to document visible evidence of disease. Eyecare physicians have also been instrumental in the development and design of specialized camera equipment needed to image an eye.

An ophthalmologist is credited with first attempting fundus photography. Although Dr. Henry Noyes considered his two negative images of the retinal vessels of a rabbit's eye to be "...very imperfectly represented...",[6] his achievement was remarkable considering the primitive equipment available in 1862. Further attempts by a number of investigators improved results, and by 1926, when a commercial model of the fundus camera was introduced, clinical fundus photography had become a practical reality.

Almost 100 years after Noyes worked on the development of fundus photography, two student doctors at Indiana University School of Medicine performed the very first human fluorescein angiogram.[7] Their success in demonstrating the flow of retinal circulation in a live person was revolutionary and heralded in a new era in ophthalmic photography. In addition to their documentary importance, ocular photographs now have a valuable diagnostic role to play.

The Role of the Eyecare Professional in Ocular Photography

Because the equipment used to photograph an eye is similar to the instruments used in a routine eye examination, many ophthalmologists are skilled in ocular photography and take their own pictures. However, most prefer to delegate this time-consuming, yet fascinating, task to others. In some practices, a photographic specialist takes all the pictures; but more often, the eyecare professionals who assist the ophthalmologist in other facets of clinical practice are selected to perform the photographic duties.

Every time a patient's vision or intraocular pressure is checked, valuable information is being gathered. Ocular photography is another way of collecting data. Instead of obtaining a numerical value, such as 20/20 or 12 mm of Hg, the information acquired is visual—a negative, slide, or print. Whatever the test, the best results are obtained when the person performing the procedure is able to elicit cooperation from the patient. Skilled eyecare professionals manage their patients well. Because of this, a competent assistant, technician, or technologist can usually become quite adept at taking pictures with a minimum amount of photographic training.

RA

The Patient as a Photographic Subject

Although ocular specimens are sometimes photographed after an eye has been removed because of disease or after death, the majority of ocular photographs are taken in a clinical setting as part of a patient examination. Some conditions are quite rare and beautiful while others, like macular degeneration, are all too common. Whether your subject has an unusual corneal dystrophy or an age-related condition, bear in mind that eye problems can be quite devastating to the patient in both visual and psychological terms. Be sensitive and never forget that your patient is a person, not a disease.

References

1. Vetter JP. Photomicrography: a translation into the vernacular, part I-the illuminating system. *J Biol Photogr*. 1987;55:81.

2. Peres M. Close-up photography and photomacrography. In: Vetter JP, ed. *Biomedical Photography*. Boston, Mass: Butterworth-Heinemann; 1992:171.

3. Vetter JP. Photomicrography. In: Vetter JP, ed. *Biomedical Photography*. Boston, Mass: Butterworth-Heinemann; 1992:156-157.

4. American Academy of Ophthalmology. Basic and Clinical Science Course: Optics, Refraction, and Contact Lenses. San Francisco, Calif; 1994:92-94.

5. Stoeckle JD and Sanchez GC. *On Seeing Medicine's Science and Art: Cure and Care, Body and Patient, the Invention of Photography and Its Impact on Learning.* Cambridge, Mass: Harvard University Press; 1989:81.

6. Mann W. History of photography of the eye. *Surv Ophthal.* 1970;15:181.

7. Alvis DL and Julian K. The story surrounding fluorescein angiography. *The Journal of Ophthalmic Photography.* 1982;5:6.

Chapter 2

Basic Photography

- The 35-mm SLR camera is preferred in scientific photography.

- The essential components of a camera are the body, aperture, lens, and shutter.

- The common characteristics of film are type, size, speed, grain, resolution, sharpness, and color balance.

- Flash illumination is recommended for patient photography.

Introduction

During the 15th century, 400 years before photography was invented, cameras were already in widespread use. It is hard to imagine that a camera without film inside could be anything but worthless, since for many of us, the word "camera" itself conjures up glossy photographic images. But a camera is actually nothing more than a room or chamber. It may be empty, contain a roll of film, or (in a legal setting) hold a sitting judge.

More than 1000 years ago, an Arab mathematician and scientist reported that when light was shone through a small hole in a tent or darkened room, an upside-down or inverted image of what was outside would be projected on the inside wall. This scientific principle became the basis for a device known as the camera obscura or "darkened room." Renaissance artists, interested in rendering objects more realistically, often used the camera obscura as a tool to improve the accuracy of their drawing. They would actually stand inside these rooms and trace the images cast on the wall, opposite the hole. By incorporating a magnifying lens, mirror, and piece of tracing glass in its design, the camera was eventually downsized from an actual room to a small box, which made it quite portable and no longer necessary (or possible) to stand inside.

In 1826, after 10 years of experimentation, the French inventor Niepce loaded a camera obscura with a bitumen-covered pewter plate and used it to obtain a stable image of the view outside his attic window. Although the result was far inferior to what we'd expect today from even the poorest quality camera, his is generally accepted as the very first photograph.

The plates used by the earliest photographers were coated with a wet, light-sensitive material that had to be exposed and processed before the coating dried. This placed new limitations on the formerly portable camera obscura since a darkroom had to be readily available whenever it was used for picture taking. Major developments in the optical and chemical sciences during the 19th century, however, helped to remedy this and other hurdles facing these pioneers. By 1888, a small camera manufactured for and marketed to the masses was introduced. The Kodak Model No. 1 was inexpensive and easy to use. With its simple design and reassuring slogan, "You press the button, we do the rest," this camera made photography the accessible and acceptable medium it is today.[1]

Cameras and Components

In order to take even a single picture, the wet-plate photographer of yesteryear had to have many pounds of necessary equipment nearby. Usually it was hauled around in a pack strapped to the photographer's back. In contrast, today's 35-mm camera operator can hold the essentials for picture taking in one hand. When it was introduced in the 1920s, the 35-mm camera was somewhat of a novelty because of its small size. Dubbed "the miniature," it was considered a toy rather than a legitimate photographic device. Today, it is the leading choice of professional photographers everywhere and an integral part of most of the specialty eye cameras used in ophthalmology.

Despite its size, a 35-mm camera can be intimidating to those unfamiliar with its various options and numerous knobs. Its many features, which contribute greatly to the ease with which a picture can be taken, also add to its seeming complexity. When stripped of its accessories, however, even the most sophisticated camera is basically a box with a hole in it. Put a magnifying glass in front of the hole and add a way to control the time that the film is exposed to light, and you have the four essential components common to all modern cameras: the body, aperture, lens, and shutter.

Camera Body

The camera body is comparable to the scleral shell of the globe—functioning primarily as a light-tight protective enclosure, shielding its contents from unwanted light. Although eyes come in a variety of colors, all are similar in size and shape. Thirty-five millimeter camera bodies, on the other hand, come in many configurations. They share a common name because the film they house measures exactly 35 mm wide. The simplest 35-mm design is an attachment camera (Figure 2-1), which is mounted to an optical device like a microscope (or fundus camera). It has very few parts. On the outside you can usually find a shutter release button, film advance lever, rewind knob, and possibly a frame counter. A take-up spool, film transport sprocket, and pressure plate (for keeping the film flat) may be all there is inside. Aiming and focusing is done with the microscope, not the camera, so no lens is needed or supplied with the camera.

The rangefinder is also a type of 35-mm camera (Figure 2-2). It is so named because of its focusing mechanism, an optical device that estimates (finds) the distance (range) to an object of interest and links this information to the camera's lens. It has everything the attachment camera has, plus one porthole for viewing the subject and another for taking the picture. The use of two different openings in one camera body means that what you see through the viewfinder is not exactly what you get on film. As a result, precise framing can be difficult with this camera.

A third type of 35-mm camera is the single lens reflex (SLR) (Figure 2-3). It has only one lens for both viewing and picture-taking. A built-in mirror sends the light entering through the lens up to the viewfinder for focusing. The mirror swings out of the way when the shutter is released, enabling an image to be formed on the film. Up until the moment of exposure, the photographer sees exactly what comes through the lens. For scientific photography, in which accuracy is essential, the SLR is preferred.

On most rangefinders the picture-taking lens is permanently connected to its body. In contrast, the lens of a SLR is usually removable. Even with its lens removed, the body of a SLR functions quite well and has been adapted for use with all types of ophthalmic cameras. In fact, some of these instruments use the viewfinder of the attached SLR as the eyepiece for the unit (Figure 2-4). If the 35-mm SLR is not mounted to the specialized eye camera, the patient's eye cannot be visualized.

Those instruments with stand-alone eyepieces (Figure 2-5) could be coupled with a simple 35- mm attachment camera, but are usually equipped with a SLR because of the multitude of useful accessories available with this body type. Photographers have come to depend on standard SLR features such as motor drives and digital timers. Performing rapid sequence angiography without the benefit of these gadgets would be unthinkable today.

The Aperture

The iris of a human eye automatically adjusts to different levels of light by varying its pupil size. A simple box camera also has a pupil, but it may be no larger than the diameter of a pin and is fixed in size. The pupil, or aperture, of the more complex 35-mm SLR camera behaves more like an eye. A mechanical (or electronic) iris diaphragm controls the amount of light entering the camera by changing the size of its aperture from small to large (Figure 2-6). The sizes of these openings are not measured in millimeters, like human pupil size, but are expressed in numbers called f-stops. Because f-stops are linked to the focal length of the lens in use, they will be covered in the section on the camera lens.

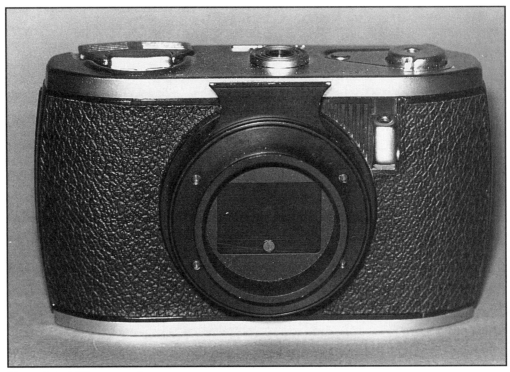

Figure 2-1. A 35-mm attachment camera.

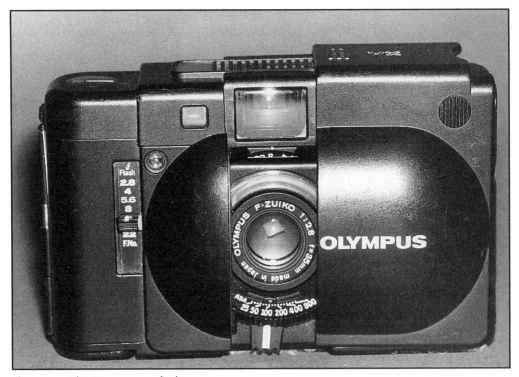

Figure 2-2. The 35-mm rangefinder.

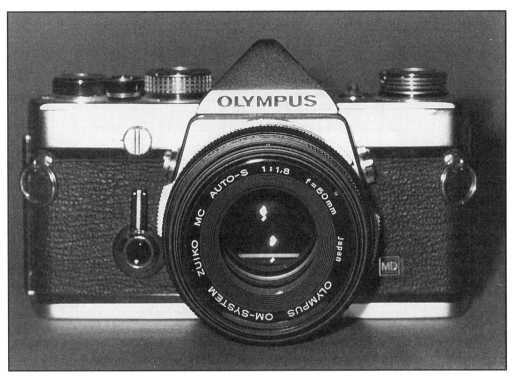

Figure 2-3. The 35-mm SLR camera.

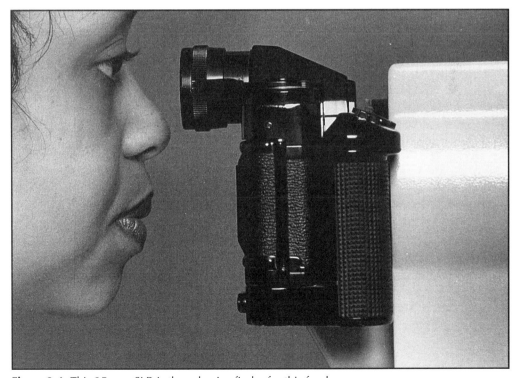

Figure 2-4. This 35-mm SLR is the sole viewfinder for this fundus camera.

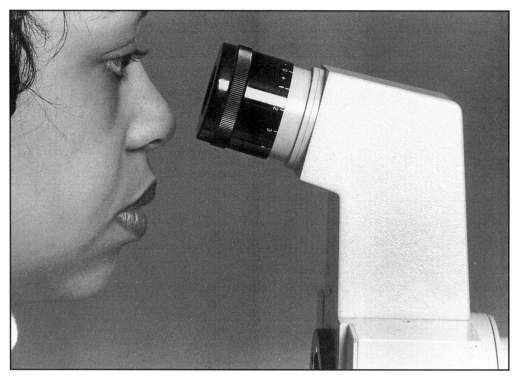

Figure 2-5. This fundus camera has an eyepiece assembly that is separate from the 35-mm SLR camera body.

The Camera Lens

In the human eye, the cornea, aqueous, lens, and vitreous all work together to refract, or bend, light so that it focuses accurately on the retina, sending nerve impulses to the brain, which "sees" the picture that is formed on the back of the eye. A camera lens also bends light to form an image of an object on the opposite side of the lens where its light-sensitive material (the film) is located. A lens is not absolutely necessary to take a picture (Figure 2-7), but it will greatly improve the sharpness of the resultant images when used.

OptA Lenses are either convex or concave. Both a normal human eye and an ordinary camera use a convex lens system to converge the light rays passing through them to form an image precisely on the retina or film. These convergent lenses bring the rays of light to a focus behind the lens **OphA** and are described as "plus" lenses. Not all eyes are normal, however. If the eyeball is too short, nearby objects cannot be seen clearly because light rays focus behind the retina. Placing a lens with the right amount of plus power in front of the eye will bend the light rays to focus on the retina. If the eyeball is too long, distant objects cannot be distinguished clearly since the focused image falls short of the retina. In this case, a minus, or concave lens, can be used to diverge the light rays after they are refracted so that they have to travel further through the eyeball to focus exactly on the retina.

The power of a pair of eyeglasses or contact lenses may be either plus or minus, depending on the patient's refractive error, but photographic lens systems have only positive power. Although the lenses of most cameras are made up of a combination of convex and concave elements mounted together and held in place in a barrel or tube, the total effect is that of a convex lens since the image is formed on the film that lies behind the lens.

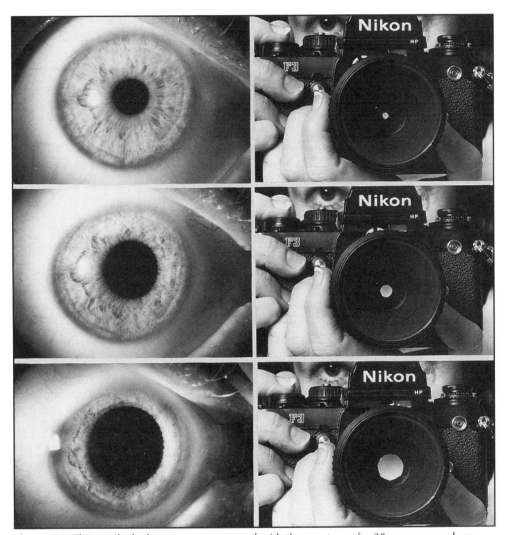

Figure 2-6. The pupil of a human eye compared with the aperture of a 35-mm camera lens.

Focusing

Focusing is the procedure of adjusting a camera lens to obtain the sharpest image of an object. One way to focus a 35-mm SLR is to rotate the focusing ring of the lens until the image in the viewfinder appears sharp. You can also focus without looking through the camera if you measure the distance between you and your subject and preset it on the lens by using the distance scale. If your subject must be recorded on film at a specific magnification (eg, 1:10) and your camera has a reproduction ratio scale, once the magnification ratio has been set, focusing is accomplished by moving the camera toward or away from the subject until it appears sharp.

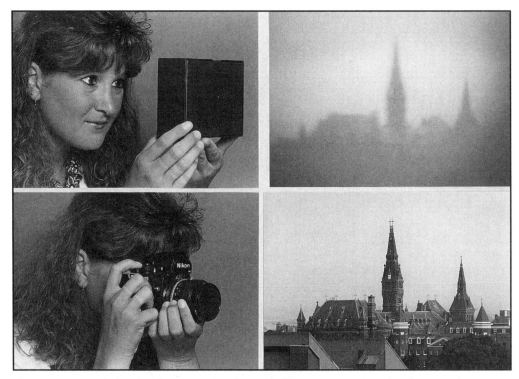

Figure 2-7. A simple lensless box camera with a pinhole aperture compared with a complex 35-mm SLR camera. Top left: A box camera. Top right: A picture taken with the box camera (Photograph by Alyce Booth). Bottom left: A 35-mm SLR in use. Bottom right: A picture taken with the SLR.

Focal Length

When parallel rays of light enter a converging lens and are brought to a focus at a point, the distance from the lens to this point is called the focal length. It is easy to calculate the focal length of a simple single-element camera lens. Focus the lens at infinity and measure the distance between the lens center and the film plane, where a sharp image of the object is found. If the distance measures 50 mm, then the camera lens has a focal length of 50 mm. If it is 100 mm, then the lens has a focal length of 100 mm.

Lenses used with 35-mm SLRs are usually made up of six or more elements. The focal length of such a complicated optical device as a multi-element lens system cannot be measured with the method described for use with a simple lens but, fortunately, this information is usually inscribed directly on the lens barrel (Figure 2-8), making such calculations unnecessary.

Although the horizontal visual field of a single eye encompasses up to 160°, the image produced by a camera equipped with a lens capable of covering only a 45° field of view is closer to what is clearly seen by a normal human eye. Despite the expansive area included within the scope of peripheral vision, full-color perception and image acuity is experienced only in the macula (the central portion of the retina). Therefore, a camera outfitted with a so-called "normal" lens covers approximately the same visual territory as the macula.

A lens with a focal length of 50 mm is considered normal for a 35-mm camera because it provides an angle of view similar to that of the macula. If a 15 mm lens was substituted and a photograph was taken from the same camera position, a much larger area of interest would be recorded, with the increased coverage obtained with its wider 110° angle of view. If, however, a very

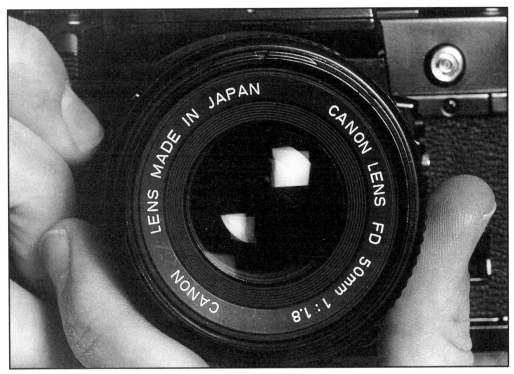

Figure 2-8. Close-up of a 35-mm camera lens with its focal length, 50 mm, inscribed on the lens barrel.

long 500 mm telephoto lens was used instead, a much smaller area would be covered by its narrower 8° field of view.

F-Stops and Lens Speed

The aperture of an ordinary 35-mm SLR camera, located in the lens assembly, can be adjusted by rotating a click-stop mechanism that moves the overlapping leaves of the diaphragm. The opening is designated by size as a standard scale of numbers called f-stops. Commonly used f-stops are 1, 1.4, 2, 2.8, 4, 5.6, 8, 11, 16, 22, 32, 45, and 64, but most modern lenses offer a range of no more than eight. Although these f-stops are written as whole numbers, they are actually fractions obtained by dividing the size of the lens opening into its focal length. The numerator is not expressed; the diameter of a lens opening measuring one-half its focal length is written as f/2 instead of 1/2.

Relative aperture, or "speed" of a lens, is a measure of the maximum capacity of a lens to transmit light. It depends on the focal length of the lens and its largest effective diameter. The largest effective diameter of a lens is obtained when the iris diaphragm is opened to its widest f-stop setting. Regardless of the number of f-stops on a given lens, its speed is a designation of its largest opening only. A very "fast" lens will have a larger opening than a "slow" lens, although the faster lens will have a smaller f-number.

With every click of the aperture ring, the amount of light entering the lens is either twice or half that of the previous f-stop. If a lens is set at f/4, "stopping down" to f/5.6 will make the opening smaller and admit only half as much light. "Opening up" a lens from f/8 to f/5.6 would double the amount of light reaching the film since the aperture is one step larger (Figure 2-9). Oftentimes, light is plentiful and the photographer may choose the f-stop from a number of acceptable

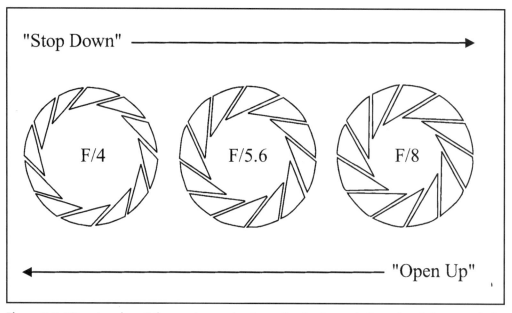

Figure 2-9. "Stopping down" the aperture makes it smaller in size and allows less light to reach the film, while "opening up" does just the opposite.

alternatives. If maximum sharpness is required, selecting the smallest aperture possible is recommended as this will increase the zone of sharp focusing (known as depth of field).

Depth of Field

The area in front of your camera within which all objects appear to be in acceptable focus is called the depth of field. Depth of field unevenly extends one-third in front and two-thirds behind the point at which you focus. The size of this zone varies with numerous factors, including focal length, f-number, and object distance.

A lens with a short focal length will provide more depth of field than a longer lens when a picture is taken from the same camera position. So, if given the choice between a 15 mm, 50 mm, or 500 mm lens of equal optical quality, and maximum sharpness is desired, the 15 mm wide-angle lens must be selected since it will yield the greatest depth of field.

As mentioned previously, selecting the smallest f-stop will also increase depth of field. When photographed with a wide-open aperture, a full-thickness corneal scar may not appear entirely focused since the shallow depth of field will not provide a sufficient zone of sharpness to adequately cover the curvature of the cornea. Sharpness can be improved if a smaller aperture is selected (Figure 2-10).

A lens focused at an object 10 ft away will yield more depth of field than if it were focused at an object 5 ft away. Because most ophthalmic photography is close-up, depth of field is severely restricted to begin with, and careful aperture selection and critical focus must take place if sharp images are expected. This can be a problem in retinal photography and fluorescein angiography, since the fundus camera's aperture is fixed and cannot be adjusted to a smaller opening to increase depth of field. The limited zone of sharp focus is especially noticeable when an elevated area of the retina is being photographed. For example, if you focus on the peak of a retinal detachment, only that part of the picture will be sharply defined. If you, instead, focus on a normal area of the same retina, the elevated area will blur while the rest of the retina is sharply

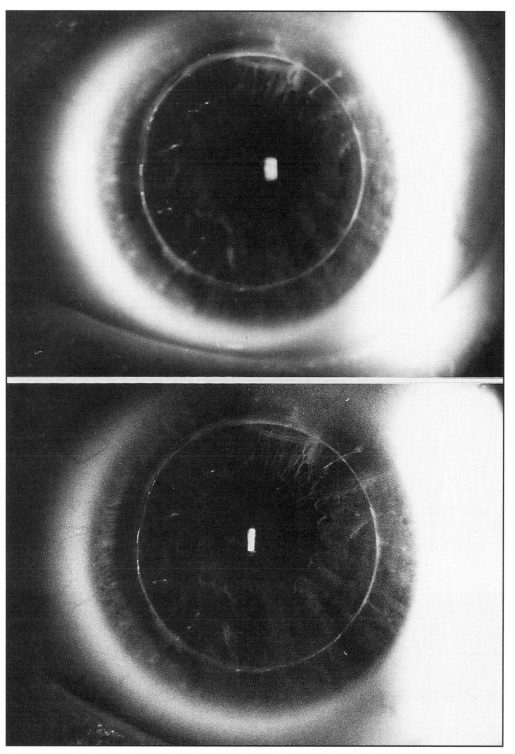

Figure 2-10. Slit lamp photographs of a corneal scar illuminated with sclerotic scatter. Top: Shot at f/14. Bottom: Shot at f/22 to enhance the depth of field.

rendered. In this case, more than one photograph will be needed to adequately capture the subject (Figure 2-11).

The Shutter

When photography was in its infancy, the available light-sensitive material was very slow to react to light. To take a picture, a photographer would simply uncover the camera's aperture, expose the film, then cover the aperture back up again. The first photograph had an exposure time of eight hours. Since those early days, film sensitivity has so greatly improved that exposures are now measured in fractions of seconds. Because it is impossible to manually uncover and cover an aperture for an exposure of less than a second, a mechanical or electric shutter capable of quickly opening and closing (like an eyelid), has been incorporated into the design of the modern camera.

The shutter of a 35-mm SLR consists of a curtain (or two) made of cloth, plastic, or metal, which, in its resting state, covers a window that lies directly in front of the film plane. In a loaded camera, unexposed film is just behind this window. When the shutter button is pressed, the curtain moves in a horizontal or vertical direction, permitting the light traveling through the lens to reach the waiting film. As the curtain sweeps across the film (Figure 2-12), different sections of the film are exposed in succession.

The length of time that the shutter is open is called shutter speed. A numbered dial, located on the camera body or lens, is set to the desired speed. Although these times are listed as whole numbers (1, 2, 4, 8, 15, 30, 60, 125, etc), they actually represent time in fractions of seconds. When you turn the dial from 1 to 500, you shorten the exposure time, since 1/500 of a second is shorter than 1 second. A slow (or low) shutter speed may be chosen to accentuate the flow of motion, but if a quick exposure is desired to freeze action, it is recommended that a fast (or high) shutter speed be selected instead (Figure 2-13).

Light-Sensitive Materials

Although technology has made it possible to record images on light-sensitive material other than photographic film, in ophthalmic photography, silver-based and color-dye emulsions are still the primary way of recording with light. Until color film was introduced, the earliest fundus photographs were taken with a limited selection of black and white film (B&W). Today, there are so many different types of films available—both color and B&W—that choosing can be difficult.

If you have a general idea of what you need, the cardboard box in which a roll of film is packaged is a wonderful resource to aid you in selecting the appropriate type of film (Figure 2-14). To the uninitiated, however, the information on the box may seem as uninterpretable as if it were written in a foreign language. An introduction to the common characteristics of film will help in your understanding of just what you need to know about this light-sensitive material.

Film Type

It is not hard to decide which film to buy while standing in the check-out line at the grocery store since your choice is usually limited to color negative film of a medium speed. Color negative film yields color negatives that must be printed onto paper (or film) to obtain a positive image. Often called "print film" because reflection prints are most popular among snapshot enthusiasts, this self-described "multi-purpose" film is not generally used in scientific photography.

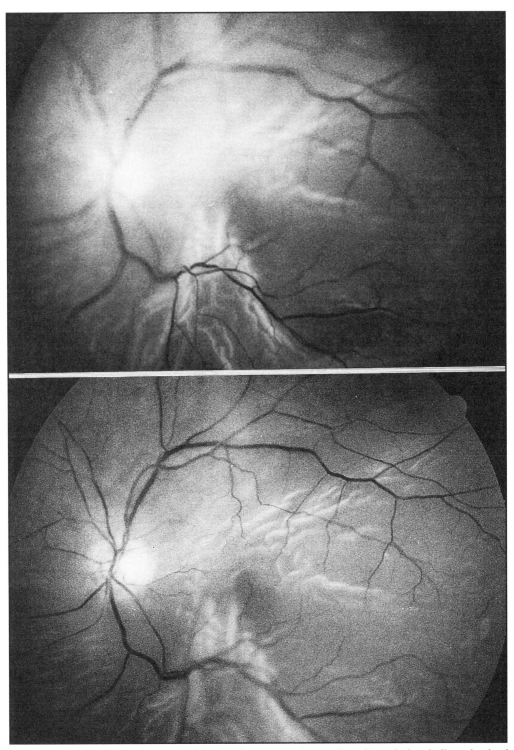

Figure 2-11. Because the aperture of the fundus camera cannot be adjusted, the shallow depth of field provided makes it necessary to carefully select the area of interest. (Note: You may need more than one picture to demonstrate the pathology if there is an elevation or depression.) Top: A detached retina in a left eye with the fundus camera focused on the apex of the detachment. Bottom: The same eye, but with the camera focused more deeply on the blood vessels in the macula area.

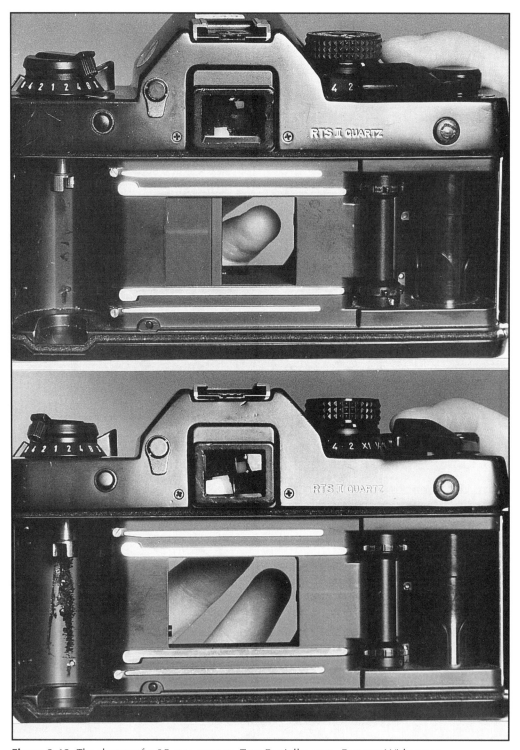

Figure 2-12. The shutter of a 35-mm camera. Top: Partially open. Bottom: Wide open.

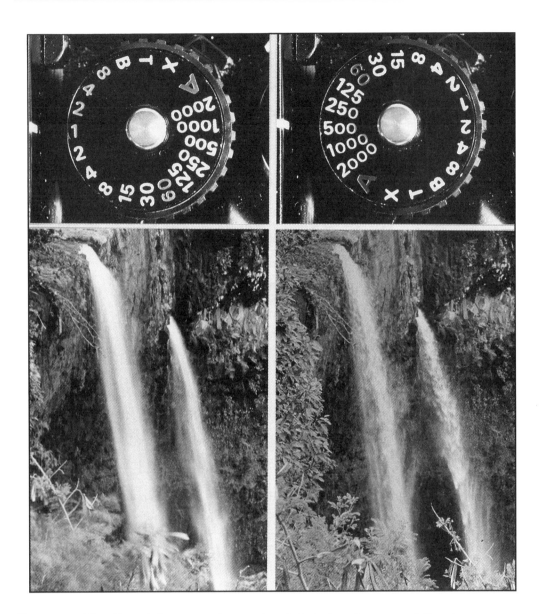

Figure 2-13. The effect of shutter speed on motion. Left: A slow shutter speed (1 sec) accentuates flow. Right: A fast shutter speed (1/500 sec) freezes motion.

Color reversal film, which yields positive color transparencies, is preferred for external eye, fundus, and slit lamp photography. Individual frames of this type of film, mounted for viewing by projection, are nicknamed "slides" because the original devices used to show the images were loaded by means of a sliding mechanism. Slides are unmatched in their versatility. Their small size make them convenient to store, and their ability to be enlarged when projected onto a big screen make them an effective teaching tool, even for large audiences.

A roll of B&W negative film yields negatives that must be printed onto paper (or film) if a positive image is desired. This type of film is used extensively in monochromatic fundus photography, fluorescein angiography, and specular microscopy. Both color transparency film and B&W negative film are easily obtained at your local camera shop.

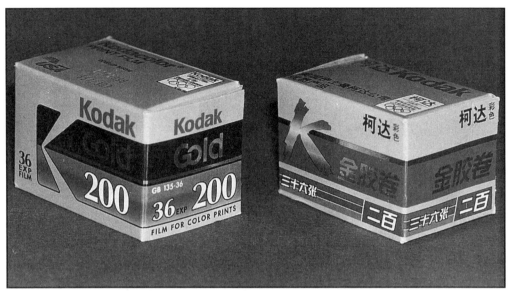

Figure 2-14. The exact same type of color negative film (ISO 200, 36 exposures) packaged for two different markets. Left: Sold in the United States of America. Right: Sold in the People's Republic of China.

Size, Speed, and Other Common Characteristics

The width of a roll of 35-mm film, including the sprocket holes, measures exactly 35 mm across, with a designated picture-taking area of 24 mm by 36 mm. Rolls of 35-mm film are generally available with 12, 24, and 36 exposures, although some films are available in 100 ft rolls containing several hundred exposures.

Like photographic lenses, all film is rated by speed, or ability to see light. Film speed is numbered by the International Standards Organization (ISO) and categorized as being either slow, medium, or fast (Table 2-1). The lower the number, the slower the film and the less sensitive it is to light. In ophthalmic photography, the 64- or 100-speed color film routinely used during fundus photography is considered to have a medium speed, while the ISO 400 B&W film used in fluorescein angiography is classified as fast.

Film speed is also a fairly good indicator of its graininess. Grain, the clumps of exposed silver or dye in B&W and color film, appears as sand-like particles in a photographic print or slide. Generally, the grain of a slow film will be smaller than the coarser, more noticeable grain structure seen in fast film (Figure 2-15), but factors other than film speed also influence the apparent graininess of a photographic image. The developer used, processing temperature, negative density, and degree of enlargement all play a role in how grain will appear in the final picture.

The overall appearance of detail in a photograph, called definition, is not solely dependent on the graininess of the film selected. A film's inherent ability to resolve fine detail (resolution) and render it with a keen edge (sharpness) will also affect the quality of the final image. Because it is not uncommon for different films of the same speed to have varying degrees of graininess, resolution, and sharpness, be careful to select the one that suits your needs.

Although our eyes (and B&W film) see a lab coat as white whether it is illuminated by the noonday sun or an ordinary household light bulb, the light emanating from these two sources is not the same color. A light bulb with a tungsten filament burns at a lower color temperature than the sun, so its light tends to be redder. Because color films vary in their ability to reproduce the color of the "white" light present in a scene, care must be taken to match the film with the type

Table 2-1

Film Speed Chart

	SLOW	MEDIUM	FAST
ISO	10	64	400
	12	80	500
	16	100	640
	20	125	800
	25	160	1000
	32	200	1250
	40	250	1600
	50	320	2000

of light being used (Figure 2-16). In ophthalmic photography, most cameras are equipped with flash units that approximate sunlight, so daylight film is recommended (rather than the type designed to be used under tungsten illumination).

The all-purpose film sold for use in recreational photography is sometimes referred to as "amateur" film because it is primarily sold for taking snapshots. Except for keeping it protected from excessive heat, this film requires no special attention. Films designated as "professional," and labeled as such, are manufactured for critical use and must be refrigerated, stored, and handled with great care. Both amateur and professional films are used in eye photography.

Flash Photography

In clinical ophthalmic photography, light from an electronic flash is used to illuminate the eye. It is reproducible, reliable, and daylight-balanced for use with a wide variety of color films and all B&W films. Before flash was introduced, patients undergoing fundus photography were subject to very long exposure times with extremely hot and bright lights. The first successful photograph of the human fundus had an exposure time of 2.5 minutes.

Like a bolt of lightning, the light emitted by a photographic flash tube is of very short duration—around 1/1000 of a second. Despite the brief burst of light from a flash, the camera's shutter must be set (Figure 2-17) to a fairly low shutter speed (or the letter "X") so that it will be fully open when the flash goes off. If it is set too high, the shutter curtain may prevent a section of the film from being exposed by blocking the incoming light (Figure 2-18). In addition, some cameras may need a synchronization cable to insure that the flash and the shutter are working together (Figure 2-19). Consult the camera's owner's manual for specific recommendations when using electronic flash.

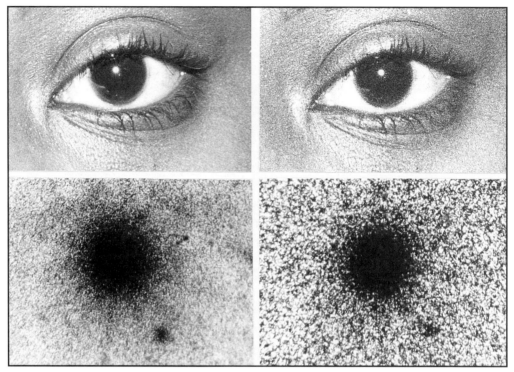

Figure 2-15. A side-by-side comparison of film graininess. Top: A positive print of a single eye enlarged from an original full-face view, shot with a "slow" film (left), and "fast" film (right) using a small flash. Bottom: An extreme close-up view of the corneal reflection from the flash (seen as a white circle in the positive photos above) in the negative of the "slow" film (left), and "fast" film (right). Because these images are microscopic enlargements of the negatives, the reflection appears black.

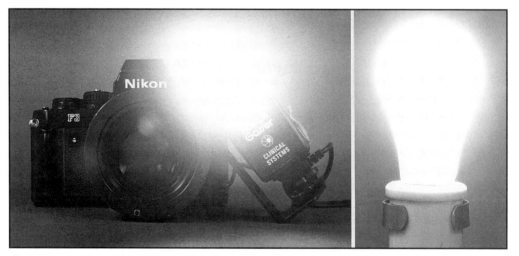

Figure 2-16. In B&W, the light from the flash (left) and light bulb (right) look the same color. A color photograph of these two sources, however, would show that each light is a different color of white. A light bulb with a tungsten filament will produce a much redder light than a gas-filled flash tube, which is balanced to match the color temperature of noonday light.

Exposure

When your finger touches the tacky side of an ordinary piece of clear tape, its impression is left behind, captured by the tape's adhesive surface. The image of your fingerprint is manifest, being readily visible. When you take a picture, the emulsion side of a piece of photographic film is also touched, but the light will not leave a readily visible impression. Instead, a latent image lies in a state of dormancy, hidden in the film's emulsion until the film is developed.

In photography, exposure is the act of subjecting a sensitized photographic material to light. Allowing too much or too little light to strike the film will create an exposure, but it won't result in a technically good image since maximum detail can be obtained only when the film is optimally exposed (Figure 2-20).

Exposure is controlled by the aperture and shutter on a 35-mm SLR camera. When a flash is used, it, too, plays an important role in determining the amount of light that will reach the film. To insure that the film is correctly exposed, select the appropriate f-stop, shutter speed, and flash output for the subject and the film in use.

Conclusion

Because they both "take pictures," it is inevitable that the camera be compared to the eye. Familiarity with the structure and function of the camera, combined with knowledge of the anatomy and physiology of the eye, will enhance your ability to serve your patients while you "see" through the eye of your camera.

Reference

1. Time-Life Books. *The Camera. Life Library of Photography.* Alexandria, Va: Time-Life Books; 1981:156.

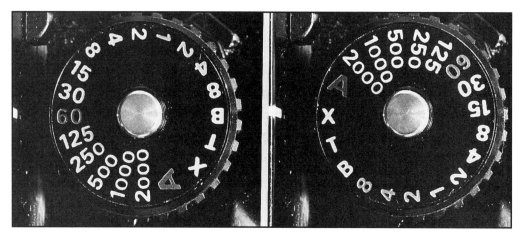

Figure 2-17. Select the shutter speed to synchronize with the flash in use. Many cameras' shutters couple with the flash at a speed of 1/60 of a second. On some cameras, setting the shutter speed dial to "x" will also synchronize the shutter with the flash.

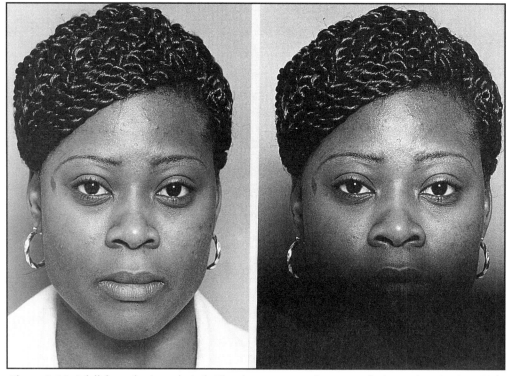

Figure 2-18. A full-face photograph. Left: The shutter was set for proper flash synchronization. Right: The shutter was set improperly for use with an electronic flash. The dark band across the bottom is where the shutter blocked the light before it struck the film.

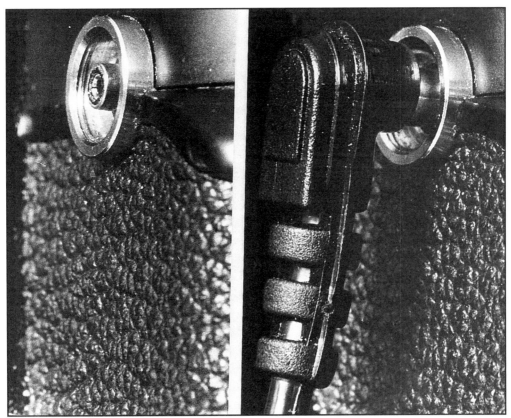

Figure 2-19. Flash synchronization chord. Left: The outlet for the flash synchronization cord. Right: The flash cord properly installed in the outlet.

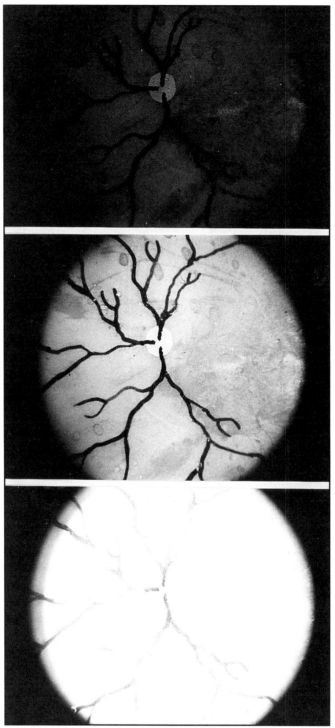

Figure 2-20. The importance of optimal exposure. Top: A positive print made from an underexposed negative will be darker than expected. Middle: A positive print made from a properly exposed negative will be just right. Bottom: A positive print made from an overexposed negative will be lighter than expected. (Note: These photos were taken of a model fundus.)

Chapter 3

The Darkroom

KEY POINTS

- The darkroom must be properly ventilated due to gases, vapors, and dust, which are produced during the developing process.

- Develop your film as soon as possible after taking the photographs.

- A data sheet suggesting solutions, dilutions, times, and temperatures is usually included with every roll of film and serves as a recipe for developing film shot under ordinary conditions.

- Film-developing chemicals include developer, stop bath, and fixer. The film is then washed and allowed to dry in a clean and dust-free environment.

- Even if you do not process your own film, familiarity with B&W developing and printing will help you become a better photographer.

The Photographer's Operating Room

A darkroom is a designated space in which light-sensitive photographic materials are handled and processed. Like the surgeon's operating room, it is a special place with a unique atmosphere, unusual equipment, and its very own set of conventions. Those who enter the darkroom have an opportunity to learn some of the more practical aspects of the craft of photography, such as exposure and composition, which can improve their general photographic skills if the lessons learned in developing and printing film are applied to actual picture-taking situations.

The first thing you may notice about a working photographic darkroom is the smell, which can be especially pungent when chemical solutions are being mixed. Having an adequate ventilation system with a supply of fresh air and an exhaust fan will help to remove most of the odor. More importantly, proper ventilation insures that the air you breathe is properly diluted of the hazardous gases, vapors, and caustic dust produced during the photographic process.

One thing that you may not notice about a darkroom is its temperature. The thermostat in an ideal darkroom will be set at or near 20°C (68°F), which is compatible with most photographic processes. This makes it possible to use stored developer, stop bath, and fixer "as is," without wasting any time heating or cooling these solutions. Because all of the liquids used in film processing must be kept to within a few degrees of the developer, the water supply in a good darkroom is also maintained at around 20°C to avoid damage to film from temperature extremes.

Another characteristic peculiar to a photographic darkroom is the lighting. You may be surprised to learn that not all photographic processes are performed in the dark. When making black and white contact prints or enlargements, a colored "safelight" is sometimes used. It is safe to use this light only if the film or paper is blind to its color, however. A color-blind material will have words like "open under proper safelight illumination" printed on the box. If the warning, "open in total darkness" appears instead, your film or paper is not safe and will be fogged when exposed to light of any color. Fog, a defect which shows up as density in processed photosensitive material and is not attributable to the action of image-forming radiation, can irreparably damage film. To protect your film from unnecessary light damage, heed the manufacturer's warning by working in total darkness and keeping your distance from any source of light.

Daylight developing tanks (Figure 3-1), which permit liquid to get in and out without admitting any light, give the photographer the option of processing film in total darkness or with the room lights on. The ingenious design of these tanks makes the darkroom superfluous when used in conjunction with a light-tight changing bag (Figure 3-2). Loading film onto the reel and into the tank takes place in the bag—all subsequent steps can be done in a lighted area.

Darkrooms are usually divided into "wet" and "dry" sides. A sink is the prominent feature of the wet side. Any time a liquid is being used, work should take place in this area. Other tasks, such as loading film onto a developing reel or exposing paper under the photographic enlarger, should be done on the dry side of the darkroom. If a single drop of water or chemical solution comes in contact with a piece of film or paper before it is processed, the undeveloped "latent" image could be ruined.

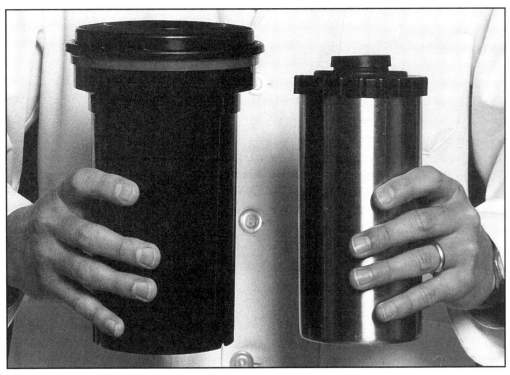

Figure 3-1. Daylight developing tanks. Left: Plastic. Right: Stainless steel.

Film Development

OphMT
RA

Until it is processed, film is susceptible to changes that can affect its latent image (Figure 3-3). A roll of color film baking inside a car's glove compartment on a hot summer day will exhibit damage from too much heat just as a roll of B&W film dropped in a mud puddle will show signs of fluid immersion. To avoid such problems from improper storage, have your film developed as soon as possible after being exposed.

Developing film is not difficult. It does require specialized equipment and photographic expertise, however, so many offices use off-site processing. The color reversal film ordinarily used in external, fundus, and slit lamp photography can be handled by your local photo-finisher. Most suitably equipped "one-hour" labs can develop and mount color slide film in about the same time it takes to complete a single angiogram.

Unless you are shooting a tremendous amount of color film and are willing and able to invest a large amount of capital in the necessary equipment, it doesn't pay to process it yourself. In addition, a few of the chemicals utilized in processing color film are hazardous and best avoided to eliminate any unnecessary exposure.[1]

The film used in angiography is ordinary B&W film, but it requires special processing to maximize the information provided by the fluorescein dye. This is not usually within the scope of your local photo-finisher's expertise and should be left to those with professional experience in ophthalmic photographic processing. A handful of qualified companies are listed under "Angiography Services" in the classified pages of some ophthalmic periodicals. For a reasonable

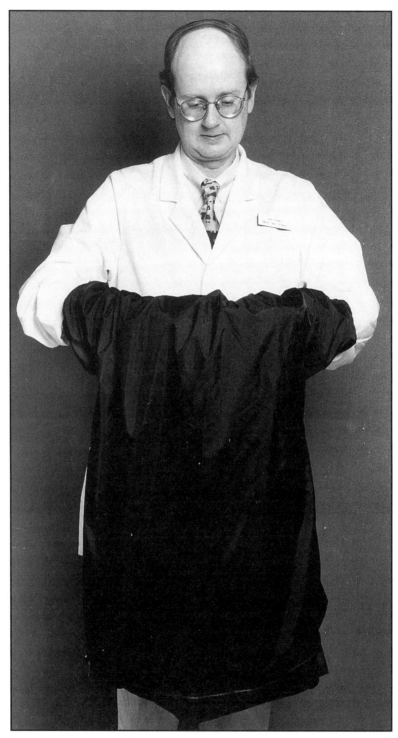

Figure 3-2. A light-tight film changing bag.

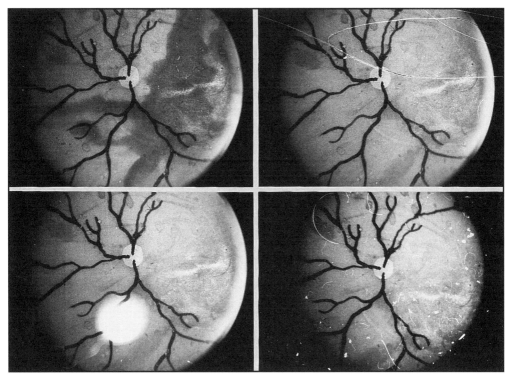

Figure 3-3. Damaged film (model eye). Top left: Water poured on film. Top right: Scratch marks. Bottom left: A drop of orange soda dried on the film. Bottom right: Dust and debris on the film.

price, they will develop, print, and return your processed film to you in just a few days.

If you work with a doctor who specializes in diseases and disorders of the retina, in-house development of B&W film is recommended to insure that a vision-threatening condition, such as macular degeneration, is promptly diagnosed and appropriately treated. Because the chemicals used in B&W processing are much less toxic than those used with color film, and the equipment investment is minimal, on-site processing of such diagnostically valuable film is advised.

Developing B&W Film

OphMT

RA

Processing B&W film is easy. To get started, you'll need an exposed roll of film, a developing tank with reel, a bottle opener, and a pair of scissors (Figure 3-4). On the dry side of the darkroom (in the dark or in a changing bag), remove the film from its cassette and wind it onto the film reel (Figure 3-5). Plastic reels load easily from the outside toward the center. In contrast, stainless steel reels are loaded from the core outward, requiring that the film be pinched (ever so slightly) between the thumb and forefinger. Too much pressure can result in localized areas of density on the negative, which appear as white crescent-shaped kink marks on the positive print (Figure 3-6).

Once the reel is loaded, place it in the tank and cover the tank with the lid. When you've accomplished this, you may turn on the room lights and proceed to the designated wet area of the darkroom.

Film processing is a lot like cooking. If you are careful and follow established procedures, the

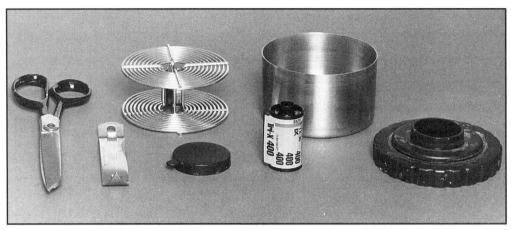

Figure 3-4. What you'll need for film development: A pair of scissors, bottle opener, film reel and tank with lid, and a roll of film.

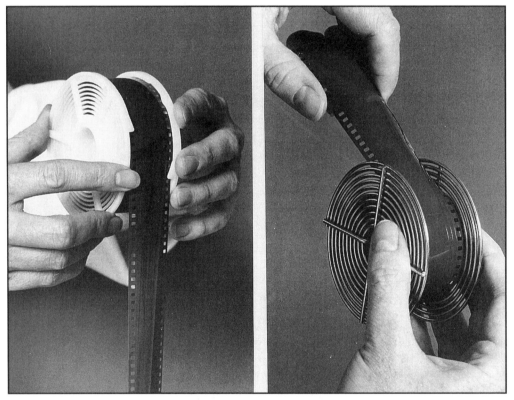

Figure 3-5. Loading film onto the reel. Left: Plastic reel. Right: Steel reel.

end result will be what you expected. A data sheet suggesting solutions, dilutions, times, and temperatures is usually included with every roll of film and will serve as a recipe for development of film shot under ordinary conditions. Unfortunately, the weak output and extremely low contrast of emitted light captured photographically during fluorescein angiography make it an extraordinary condition. Because of this, the film must be developed with a vigorous high-contrast devel-

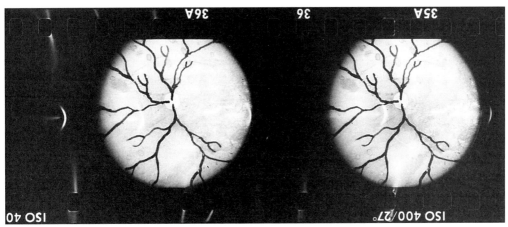

Figure 3-6. Kink marks in the film, shaped like moons or arrow heads, result when the film is bent excessively while loading a steel reel (A model fundus was used).

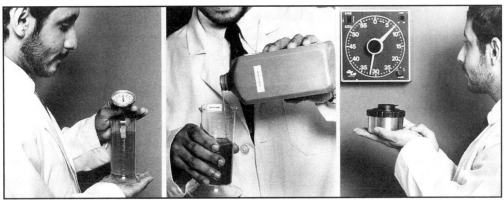

Figure 3-7. Precision is required when measuring the temperature and volume of the solutions used in processing film as well as the length of time during which the various steps take place.

oper not usually listed on the data sheet. If you are not sure which developers are compatible with the film and camera you are using, contact the fundus camera's manufacturer for their suggestions or ask an experienced ophthalmic photographer to make a recommendation.

After deciding which developer and development recipe to use, gather and assemble all the ingredients and necessary utensils before beginning. A watch or clock is needed to measure time, a thermometer to check the temperature, and graduated cylinders for accurately measuring the volume of the solutions (Figure 3-7).

Arrange four solution-filled graduates from left to right (Figure 3-8) in the order of their use: The first graduate will contain developer, a solution used to amplify the film's latent image. The second will contain a stop bath, which halts the action of the developer. The third container will hold the fixer, which clears the film of unexposed silver and renders it insensitive to light. The fourth container should hold water (or some other washing agent) to clear the film of all the previous chemicals.

After you have checked to be sure that the developer is the proper temperature and set the clock for the appropriate development time, you are ready to begin. With the tank slightly tilted, pour the developer into its spout as quickly as possible without spilling (Figure 3-9). Start the timer when the tank is full of developer, tap the tank once or twice (to eliminate air bubbles),

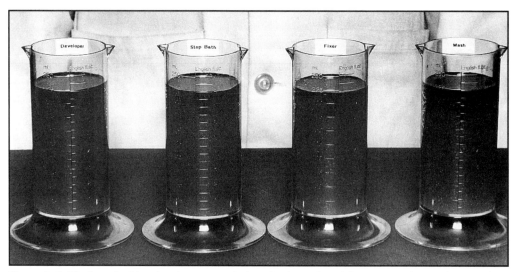

Figure 3-8. Black and white development solutions in the order of their use. Left to right: Developer, stop bath, fixer, and wash. (Note: To make the solutions more visible, colored liquid was used instead of actual photographic liquids, which are normally clear.)

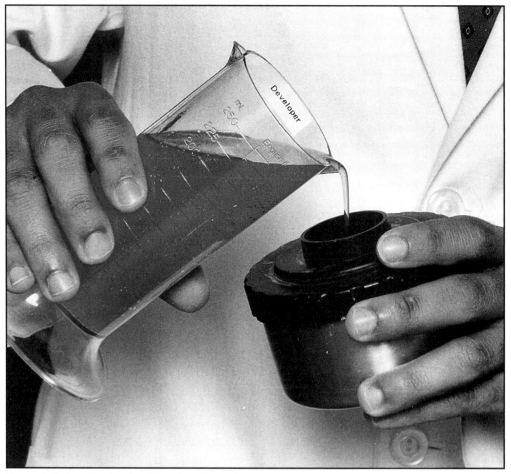

Figure 3-9. Pouring the developer into the tank.

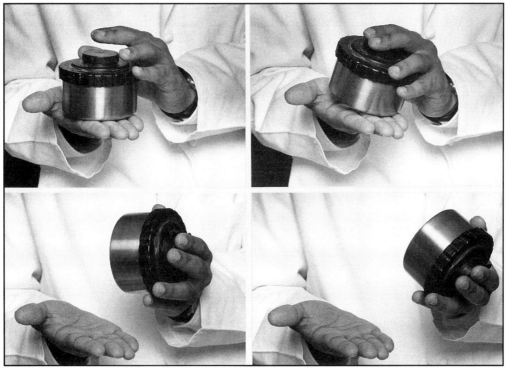

Figure 3-10. Agitating a steel tank using the inversion method.

place the cap on the lid, and agitate as recommended on the data sheet. A solution-filled stainless steel tank is agitated by rotating it in a circular direction and/or inverting it (Figure 3-10). A plastic tank has a stirring rod. Unless the manufacturer specifies a certain type of agitation, different methods may be used with equally positive results.

When the required time for development has elapsed, pour out the exhausted solution. Quickly pour the contents of the second graduate into the tank and agitate continuously. This graduate contains an acidic solution called "stop bath," which is used to halt the action of the developer. Sometimes ordinary tap water is used instead. When the required time is up, pour out the stop bath and discard, unless a reusable type is being used.

Fill the tank with the fixer contained in the third graduate. Fixer will make the developed images on the film permanent. It, too, usually requires constant agitation for optimum results and may be reusable. After fixing, film can be safely exposed to light. What you'll see is a negative image of what you saw through your camera's viewfinder. Anything that was white (or light) in the scene will appear black (or dark) on film, and whatever was black will be seen as white. Tonally, a photographic negative of a person is an obvious opposite (Figure 3-11), but a negative from a fluorescein angiogram is not as easily perceived as such (Figure 3-12).

To insure its permanence, film must be washed properly and allowed to dry in a clean and dust-free environment. Once dry, the roll of film should be cut into strips and placed in protective pages, sleeves, or envelopes, where it is safe from dust, scratches, fingerprints, and other hazardous elements or environmental pollutants.

The film itself may be the end product of fluorescein angiography if the interpreting physician is adept at reading negatives. For those physicians (and photographers) unaccustomed to seeing bright fluorescent dye as black or are disconcerted by the negative representation, a positive print should be provided.

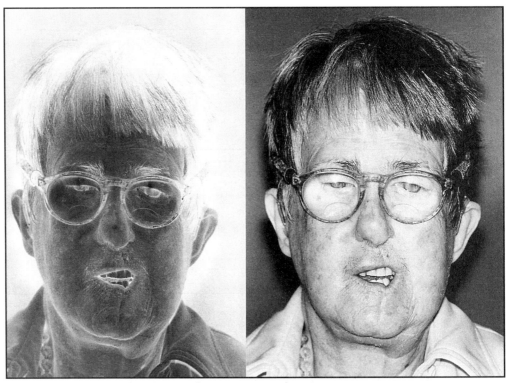

Figure 3-11. An image of a person. Left: A negative. Right: A positive.

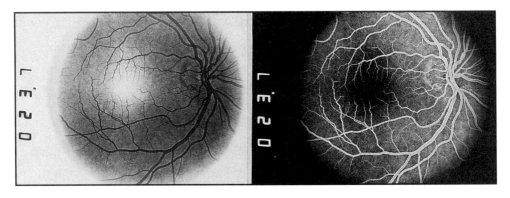

Figure 3-12. An image of fluorescein dye in the retinal circulation. Left: A negative. Right: A positive.

Printing

Contact Prints

A contact print is made by placing the negatives in direct contact with a sheet of photographic paper (or transparency film) and then exposing it to white light. This may be done with a printing frame, mechanical printer, or an enlarger adapted for use as a contact printer. Excellent results can be obtained regardless of the type of contact printer used. The basic requirements are the same: The

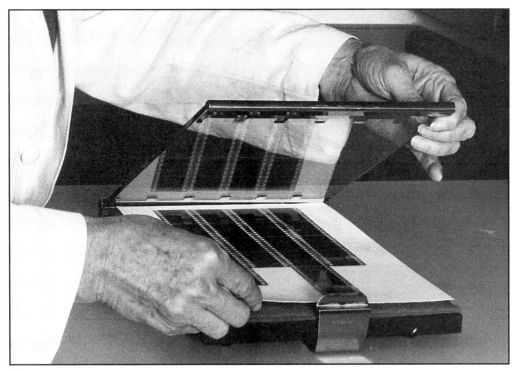

Figure 3-13. A contact printer in use.

negatives and paper must be held tightly together (Figure 3-13) during exposure to the printing light.

After development, the images on the sheet of paper are negatives of negatives (or positives), which represent the true tonal relationships of the subjects that were photographed (Figure 3-14). In most cases, a contact print of a fluorescein angiogram will provide sufficient information for interpretation if viewed under adequate magnification. Occasionally, however, an enlargement is desired.

Projection Prints

In the early days of photography when all prints were made by the contact method, if you wanted a big picture you needed to use a camera large enough to hold a negative the exact same size as the desired print. Today, with the help of a photographic enlarger (Figure 3-15), large prints can be made from even very small negatives.

An enlarger is a photographic device used to make prints by projection. Depending on the projection printer's optical components and mechanical characteristics, the distance between its lens and baseboard can be set to make prints smaller than, the same size as, or larger than the negative being printed (Figure 3-16). Since most projection prints are enlarged, the projection printer is often called an enlarger.

In projection printing, the negative itself never touches the sheet of paper as it does in contact printing. Instead, it is placed between the enlarger's light source and a lens. The lens projects the image from the negative onto the paper below. It is a kind of camera in reverse. Focusing is accomplished by adjusting the distance between the negative and the lens.

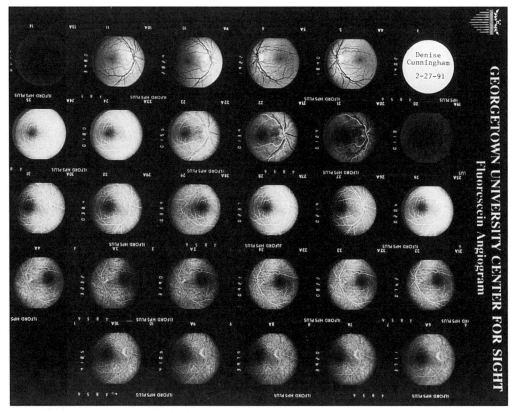

Figure 3-14. A positive contact sheet.

Conclusion

In order to skillfully perform as an ophthalmic photographer in the clinic, it is not necessary for you to become a technical expert in the darkroom. Having knowledge about and familiarity with B&W film development and printing, however, will enhance your ability to diagnose problems related to the photographic process or malfunctioning camera equipment. Recognizing the problem is often the first step to finding a solution.

Reference

1. Shaw S. *Overexposure: Health Hazards in Photography*. Carmel, Calif: The Friends of Photography, Inc; 1983:182.

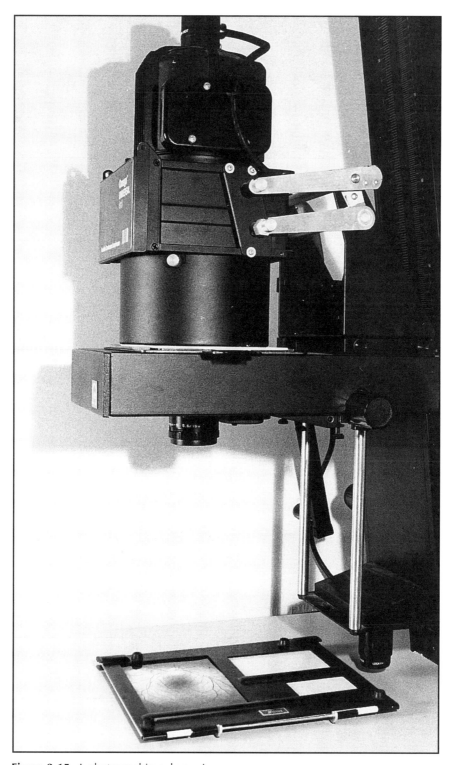

Figure 3-15. A photographic enlarger in use.

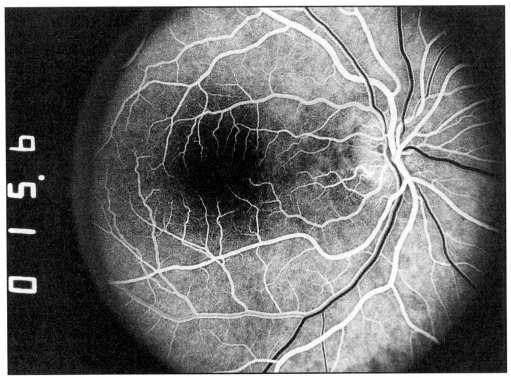

Figure 3-16. An enlargement (compare with Figure 3-14).

Chapter 4

External Eye Photography

- Establish standard photographic views to eliminate the guesswork in external eye photography.

- Use a photographic requisition form to simplify the external eye photography process.

- Select the simplest equipment that satisfies your photographic needs.

Purpose

Photography has long provided physicians with an excellent means of producing accurate and informative clinical records. A dermatologist might rely on a photograph to demonstrate the size, location, color, and texture of a skin lesion, while a plastic surgeon may use before-and-after views to evaluate the success of a new surgical technique. Ophthalmologists, trained in both the medical management and surgical treatment of diseases and disorders of the eye, may make extensive use of the camera to record both medical and surgical changes in the outward appearance of their subject—the human eye. Optometrists may likewise use photographs to document ocular findings.

Indications

The optometric or ophthalmic setting in which you work will dictate the kinds of external ocular conditions that you are most likely to photograph. If you work in the eye department of a big city hospital, some of the problems you see, no doubt, will be directly related to trauma. If your doctor specializes in pediatrics, the eyes of children with abnormalities of the ocular muscles will be your most common subject. Pre-operative photographs documenting the drooping of a patient's upper eyelid may be routinely obtained if your employer is an oculoplastic surgeon. Virtually anything deemed interesting or valuable to the physician may be recorded if the patient is willing to be photographed.

Patient Orientation and Education

When a patient agrees to be photographed, it is not usually necessary to explain the function of the camera before you begin shooting. In today's world, almost everybody has had their picture taken and has seen (and probably used) a camera. The focus of patient orientation during external eye photography is more about the purpose of the photographic session than on the equipment being used. Patients want to know why pictures are being taken of their eyes. Are they for documentation, education, or publication? Some patients may be perfectly willing to be photographed for recording their own progress but may strenuously object to the inclusion of a picture of their eye in a medical school lecture or as an illustration in a medical journal. If the intent is to circulate or publish an image in which the patient can be recognized, then permission must be obtained from that patient or guardian. The use of a written consent form is recommended (FORM 4-1).

Patients want to know their specific role as a photographic subject and what is required of them. You will hear such questions as, "How many pictures do you need? How long will this take? What do I do? Where should I look?" and "Do you want me to smile?" If you and your physician have established a specific number and type of photographs to be taken of the ocular conditions you are most likely to encounter, you can answer your patient's questions with confidence and certainty. For example, a patient with a cranial nerve palsy might undergo a standard motility series. This series usually consists of a head shot plus pictures of both eyes in primary position, upgaze, downgaze, looking left, and looking right. Without hesitation, you can say to the patient with the nerve palsy, "I'm going to take six pictures of your eyes, and it will take about three minutes of your time." Knowing what to expect can help relieve a patient's anxiety.

What the Patient Needs to Know

- These pictures will be part of your medical record.
- With your written consent, these photographs may also be used in medical teaching, education, research, or published in professional journals or medical books.
- Do not turn your head or body. Only your eyes should move.
- This camera uses a flash, which will fire for every picture.
- You are not being x-rayed.

Physician's Orders

Once a protocol has been instituted for external eye photography, the actual picture taking is simplified since the guesswork is eliminated. In our practice, a variety of standard series have been established to cover most situations and diagnoses (Figure 4-1). A facial deformity may warrant extensive photography as covered in an "eye plastic series." The "nine positions of gaze series" best demonstrates a deviation from normal position and may be chosen for a patient with strabismus (Figure 4-2). To document a blowout fracture, an "orbital series" (which includes a worm's eye view [Figure 4-3]) might be ordered. If you are already using standard views but they are different from those listed here, don't be alarmed. The type and number of views that you select as standard should be customized to fit your specific clinical needs.

If your standard views are printed on a requisition form (FORM 4-2), the photographic process is simplified in two ways. First, the ordering physician can easily check or circle the desired views. Second, you have a handy checklist of exactly what needs to be done. Providing a space on your form for the physician to depict the problem area is also helpful if the pathology is subtle or hard to find. A simple sketch saves words and clarifies descriptions.

The Photographic Plan

Once it has been decided what is needed, you must plan the photographic session. For example, if you are asked to take an "eye plastic series," there are seven different views required, but only three changes in camera-to-patient distance are needed to obtain the appropriate magnification (Figure 4-4). The most logical plan is to begin farthest from the patient with the head shot, take a few steps forward shooting both eyes together, and finish by moving close enough to the patient to obtain the desired single-eye views. It is also more natural to start at a distance from your subject and move closer as necessary, especially when working with a new patient. When given sufficient space to adjust to unfamiliar surroundings, a patient is more likely to relax and cooperate during the session.

Equipment

With the proper equipment, many layers of the eye—from the cornea to the choroid—can be imaged and recorded in a living subject. Some instruments, like the fundus camera, are complicated pieces of machinery, while others, like the external eye camera, are modern versions of the

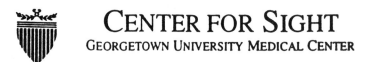

CENTER FOR SIGHT
GEORGETOWN UNIVERSITY MEDICAL CENTER

Photographic Consent Form

1.   I, _____ , consent to having photographs taken of me, or parts of my body, in connection with the medical services which I am receiving from my physician, Dr.

2.   The photographs shall be used for medical records and, if in the judgement of my physician, medical research, education, or science will benefit from their use, may be published or used in other ways deemed appropriate.

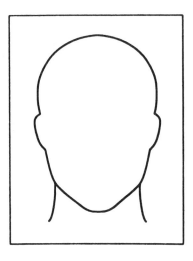

3.   I specifically understand that I shall not be identified by name if these photographs are published.

4.   The aforementioned photographs may be modified or retouched in any way that my physician may consider desirable.

FORM 4-1. A written photographic consent form.

External Eye Photography Standard Series

☐ **Eye Plastic Series**
Head Shot (1:10)
Both Eyes (1:4)
• Primary Position
• Upgaze
• Downgaze
Each Eye (1:2)
• Primary Position

☐ **Orbital Series**
Eye Plastic Series
Worm's Eye View (1:4)

☐ **Nine Positions of Gaze**

☐ **Motility Series**
Head Shot (1:10)
Both Eyes (1:4)
• Primary Position
• Upgaze
• Downgaze
• Looking Left
• Looking Right

☐ **Ptosis Series**
Both Eyes (1:4)
• Primary Position
• Upgaze
• Downgaze

☐ **Other** _____

Figure 4-1. A sample external eye photography standard series.

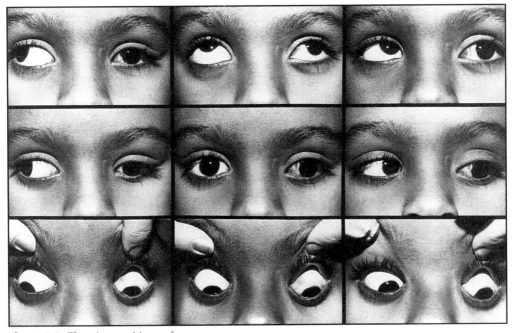

Figure 4-2. The nine positions of gaze.

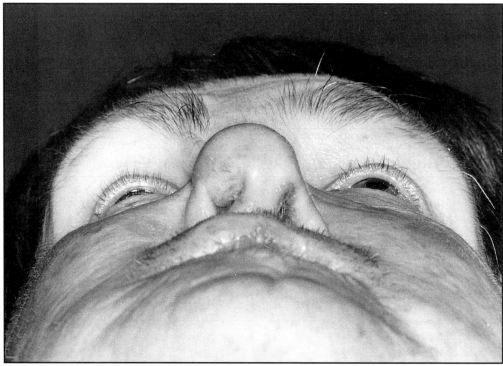

Figure 4-3. A "worm's eye view" is accomplished by having the patient tilt her head back while looking up. It may be necessary for the photographer to kneel down directly in front of the patient to view the eye as a worm might.

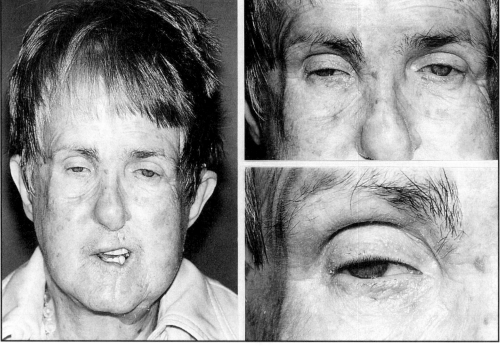

Figure 4-4. Three views of the subject taken at different camera-to-patient distances using a 105 mm lens on a 35-mm camera. Left: Position #1: head shot (1:10), taken at about 4 ft from the subject. Top right: Position #2: both eyes together (1:4), taken at about 2 ft from the subject. Bottom right: Position #3: a single eye (1:2), taken at a position a little more than a foot from the subject.

CENTER FOR SIGHT
GEORGETOWN UNIVERSITY MEDICAL CENTER

Anterior Segment Photography

Date: _____

Name: _____ DOB: _____ Age: _____ Sex: _____

Physician: _____ Referring Physician: _____

Address: _____

Ocular
Diagnosis: _____ ICD.9 Code(s) _____

Reason for Photos: _____

External Eye Photography:

☐ **Eye Plastic Series**
Head Shot (1:10)
Both Eyes (1:4)
• Primary Position
• Upgaze
• Downgaze
Each Eye (1:2)
• Primary Position

☐ **Orbital Series**
Eye Plastic Series
Worm's Eye View (1:4)

☐ **Nine Positions of Gaze**

☐ **Motility Series**
Head Shot (1:10)
Both Eyes (1:4)
• Primary Position
• Upgaze
• Downgaze
• Looking Left
• Looking Right

☐ **Ptosis Series**
Both Eyes (1:4)
• Primary Position
• Upgaze
• Downgaze

☐ **Other** _____

Slit Lamp Photography:

OD   OS

Eye(s)	Illumination
☐ OD	☐ Diffuse
☐ OS	☐ Direct
☐ OU	☐ Indirect

Specular Microscopy:

Eye(s)	# of Cells
☐ OD	OD OS
☐ OS	
☐ OU	

FORM 4-2. A photographic requisition form designed to be used for external eye and slit lamp photography, as well as specular microscopy.

simple box camera. Don't be fooled by the fast lenses, speedy motor drives, and other gadgets that dress up today's external eye cameras. When stripped of their non-essential trappings, they are still basically light-tight boxes with holes in them.

The Camera

A 35-mm SLR camera is generally used in external eye photography because it is equipped for coupling with an electronic flash and the lenses are interchangeable. The flash eliminates the need to use hot incandescent lights, and a comfortable working distance is more easily established with a longer-than-normal lens.

The Lens

A lens with a 50 mm focal length is considered "normal" for a 35-mm camera. It is a good general purpose lens designed to focus clearly on objects from about 18 inches to infinity, but not well-suited for close-up work where you want to fill the frame with a small subject. If you try to photograph a single eye with an ordinary 50 mm lens, you'll find you cannot get close enough to the patient to frame the eye and still maintain sharp focus.

Adding supplementary lenses, extension tubes, a bellows, or a lens reversing ring will allow close-up photographs to be taken with a normal lens, but these attachments also complicate things. An easier way is to employ a special close-up macro lens, which is designed to photograph small subjects (like the human eye) tightly framed and clearly focused at less than 18 inches. Although a 50 mm macro lens could be used, its short working distance makes it an impractical choice when photographing live subjects. It may be too close for comfort for some patients. Converting to a lens with a longer focal length allows the subject to be framed and focused at a less intrusive distance (Figure 4-5). The additional working space also affords the photographer greater control over flash placements.

The Light

The flash has revolutionized ophthalmic photography. Before its invention, some of the earliest retinal photographs were taken by the light of a carbon arc lamp. The heat from the light and the long exposure time made the process so uncomfortable that the patient's cornea had to be anesthetized with topical cocaine. Today, a burst of light from the camera's flash lasts just a fraction of a second—all that is needed to sufficiently light the inner eye. The tube of the flash is filled with an inert gas (usually xenon), which does not conduct electricity. When the camera's shutter is released, electrical energy flows through it as a high intensity current, causing the gas to glow brightly, lighting up the eye. All but the most photophobic patients have little difficulty handling its intensity.

Both the fundus and slit lamp cameras use large flash units with enough current to kill by electric shock. On some older models, you can actually hear the hum of raw power surging through their capacitors. An equally powerful (and expensive) studio flash, the kind used in commercial photography, could be adapted for use in external eye photography, but such a potent source is unnecessary, and its use is ill advised given the size of the reflection it creates when used with a "soft box" (Figure 4-6). Fortunately, a flash capable of producing a high intensity source of light for a very short duration does not need to be large. In fact, most of the small amateur units on the market today are superior to the larger studio models when a highly reflective object, like a patient's eye, is the subject.

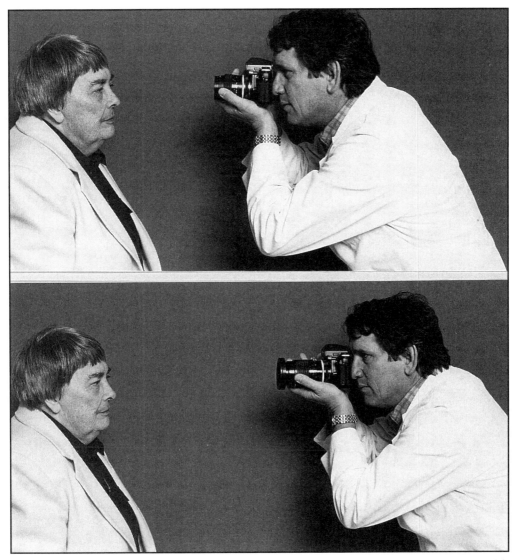

Figure 4-5. The camera-to-subject distance when photographing both eyes together at 1:4 (1/4 life size). Top: Using a 50 mm normal lens. Bottom: With a 105 mm telephoto lens.

Because the cornea is highly polished, light from any flash will reflect off its surface and be unavoidably recorded on film. To keep this reflection from obscuring any underlying pathology, it is best that a flash with the smallest reflector be used. Two different types of flashes, the point source and the ring light (Figure 4-7), are commonly used in medical photography. Although both produce a small reflection (Figure 4-8), the point source is more versatile. The ring light encircles the camera lens, and its reflection will always appear in the middle of the cornea if the eye is centered. With an adjustable bracket, a point source flash can be rotated around the lens and placed in a more desirable position (Figure 4-9).

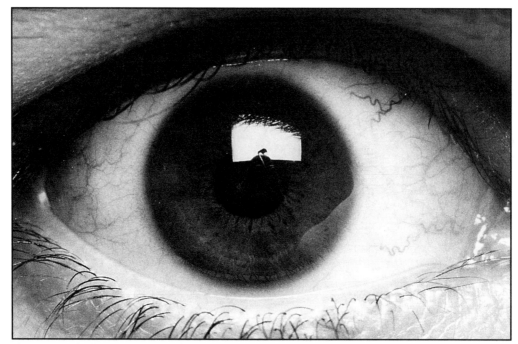

Figure 4-6. The large corneal reflection of the light source from a studio flash equipped with a "soft box."

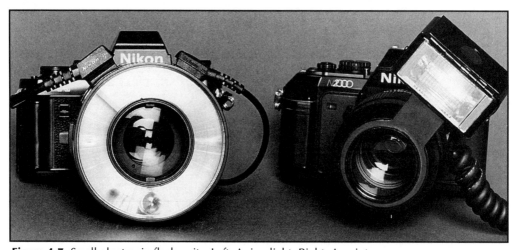

Figure 4-7. Small electronic flash units. Left: A ring light. Right: A point source.

The Film

The glow from an electronic flash has approximately the same color composition as the light emitted by the noonday sun. Since most color films are made to give accurate color in normal outdoor scenes, a daylight-balanced film is recommended for external eye photographs taken with a flash. The same medium speed color reversal film (slides) used in fundus photography may be used for external photos if the flash is sufficiently powered. Remember, for increased depth of field, select film with the slowest possible speed that will allow you to take advantage of your camera's smaller lens openings.

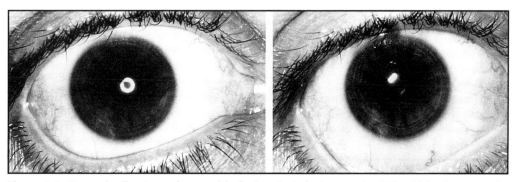

Figure 4-8. Corneal reflections of a portable flash unit. Left: From a ring light. Right: From a point source.

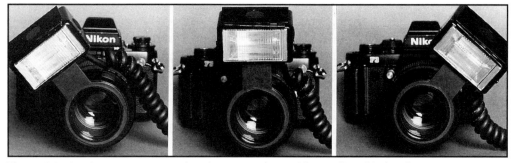

Figure 4-9. A point source mounted to the camera lens with an adjustable bracket.

When choosing a film for external eye photography, consider your subject. If your photographs include many full-face views or eyelids, using the type of film appropriate for photographing the retina may be unacceptable if it records skin tones unnaturally. Because different types of color film represent colors with slight and distinct color differences, it makes sense to try a number of different films before settling on one particular type .

Conclusion

The ability of color slide film to provide an accurate and detailed representation of the eye and adjacent structures makes it an ideal film for external eye photography. A simple arrangement consisting of a hand-held 35-mm camera, long lens, and portable flash is recommended for this basic ocular procedure.

Chapter 5

Fundus Photography

KEY POINTS

- Fundus photographs provide accurate visual records of the inner eye.

- All pathological conditions of the fundus do not require photographs for proper diagnosis and treatment.

- A fundus camera consists of a main camera unit, base assembly, and power supply.

- For documentation of most intraocular structures, daylight color positive transparency (slide) film is used.

- Some intraocular structures (such as the choroid, retinal vasculature, and nerve fiber layer) are better appreciated when photographed with black and white film.

- If the camera is too far from or too close to the eye, or not centered on the pupil, unwanted light reflections will appear in the picture.

`OptT`

`OphT`

`RA`

Purpose

A fundus is the bottom, back, or base of a hollow organ. If you've worked with eyes, you've probably heard the term "ocular fundus" used to describe the inside of the eye. The word fundus is not unique to the fields of optometry and ophthalmology. You may be surprised to learn that gastroenterologists, gynecologists, and urologists can also point to the fundus of their patients' stomach, uterus, or bladder.

To examine the ocular fundus, an eye specialist uses an ophthalmoscope or a slit lamp biomicroscope with a funduscopic lens, but a special camera (Figure 5-1) is needed when high quality pictures are expected. Although photographs have been taken successfully with cameras attached to both indirect ophthalmoscopes and photo slit lamps, a fundus camera is recommended for this task.

Taking pictures with a fundus camera is called fundus photography. It is the most basic form of inner eye photography. Unlike diagnostic fluorescein angiography (discussed in Chapter 6), it is purely documentary in nature, providing the physician with an objective record of how things looked inside the eye at the moment the picture was taken. Although optometrists and ophthalmologists still use colored pencils to sketch out their clinical observations, fundus photography with color film is preferred when the exact size, shape, or appearance of an intraocular lesion must be recorded.

Some inner ocular structures and conditions show enhanced contrast and are better appreciated (Figure 5-2) when photographed with B&W film (instead of color), using colored light, called "monochromatic" illumination. Monochromatic illumination is achieved when a filter of a single (mono) color (chrom) is used to change the light (illumination) shining into the patient's eye by altering its wavelength. Since green and blue filters are standard accessories on fundus cameras used for fluorescein angiography, these two colors are commonly selected for monochromatic photography. Convenience alone is not the only reason for using green or blue light. Green light is an excellent choice for demonstrating retinal vascular changes, while blue light provides optimal visualization of vitreoretinal interface abnormalities. If a red filter is added, choroidal disturbances may be highlighted as well.

`OptT`

`OphT`

`RA`

Indications

For scientific accuracy, high quality photographs of the fundus are generally superior to an artistic rendering, but not all pathological conditions of the inner eye need to be photographed. Many diseases and disorders of the retina, although interesting subjects, do not require photographic documentation in order for the physician to diagnose and treat them. While a single picture of a choroidal nevus may prove indispensable in monitoring growth, extensive survey photographs of a diabetic patient with a single microaneurysm are probably not valuable.

`OphT`

`RA`

Patient Education and Orientation

Fundus photography is more interesting to the person taking the pictures than to the patient being photographed. The photographer has the opportunity to view living tissue in vivo, while the patient gets blasted with light. If you've never been dilated and photographed yourself, have it done. An empathetic photographer who has gained some insight by experiencing the process is

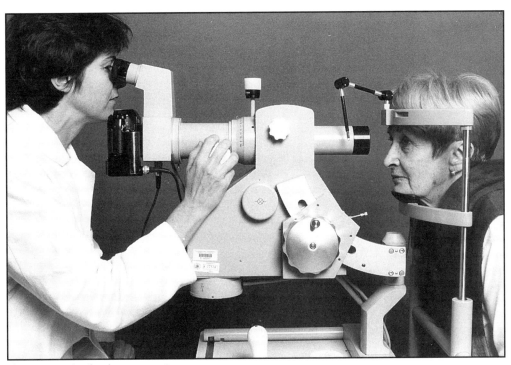

Figure 5-1. The fundus camera in use.

better able to appreciate just how difficult it can be for the patient.

If this is the patient's first experience as the subject of fundus photography, he or she must be told what you are doing and what you expect him or her to do during the photo session. You might begin by saying, "I'm going to start with your right eye, Ms. Smith. Please take your glasses off, put your head in the face rest, and follow this light when I move it." Take the mystery out of the procedure by telling patients in advance that they "may see colors" after the flash goes off. Because the room is dark, the lights are bright, and the patient is dilated, warn the patient before you touch him or her to hold an eyelid or move the head forward.

Physician's Orders

The use of a requisition form, filled out by the ordering physician, is recommended for all types of clinical photography. A form designed specifically for posterior segment work (FORM 5-1) should include space for the diagnosis and description of the area of interest, as well as a place to illustrate any pertinent or unusual findings.

Photographic Fields of View

When you look through the ocular of a fundus camera aimed directly into the eye of a patient looking straight ahead, the macula will be in your sight. If you ask the patient to look just a little bit toward his or her nose, the disc will appear. You may need to reposition the camera slightly, but when the macula and optic nerve are your only subjects, camera movement is minimal. Shifting the

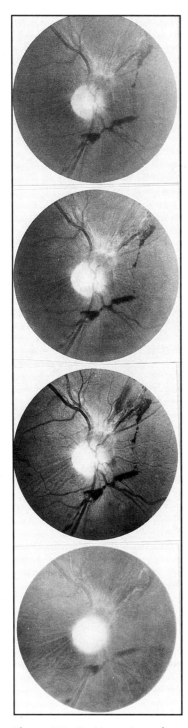

Figure 5-2. Positive prints of an eye with proliferative diabetic retinopathy made from original B&W negatives. Top: No filter used. Second from top: Blue filter used. Third from top: Green filter used. Bottom: Red filter used.

camera's joystick from left to right, or back and forth just a little bit is usually all it takes to frame these ocular landmarks.

If you must venture beyond the posterior pole, however, both the patient's eye and the fundus camera must be moved. In most cases, verbal instructions or a fixation device (Figure 5-3) will be sufficient to elicit adequate eye movement from your patient. Swings and tilts of the camera, allowing the superior, inferior, nasal, and temporal retina to be visualized, are obtained by adjusting the appropriate knobs on the instrument. By combining eye and camera moves, even peripheral areas of the retina can be photographed.

Patients enrolled in clinical research involving the inner eye may be required to undergo fundus photography, including views of their peripheral retina.

The protocol for a landmark study on diabetic retinopathy specified seven overlapping fields to be photographically mapped out for review, evaluation, and classification.[1] Although the research only concerned diabetic retinopathy, these photographic views, called the seven standard photographic fields, have been incorporated as part of many subsequent studies of retinal disease and should be familiar to all those who perform fundus photography (Figure 5-4).

The seven standard fields were designed for use with a fundus camera that imaged 30° of the retina (Figure 5-5). As wider angle cameras became available, these fields were sometimes modified by investigators to make use of the increased area of coverage (Figure 5-6). Sometimes the number of necessary photographs was reduced, but other times, because the panoramic view provided by the wide-angle camera also made it possible to photograph diseases that affect the far periphery of the fundus, the standard fields were expanded to include more than seven.

If peripheral fundus photography is part of your repertoire, then you know that it is not always possible to get clear pictures when your camera is positioned at an extreme angle. This is due to astigmatism, which is introduced by the angle of the fundus camera in relation to the patient's crystalline lens. Some cameras have a device, called an astigmatism corrector, for reducing this obliquely induced astigmatism (Figure 5-7), which often improves the view. Maximum sharpness is obtained by moving its dial until the subject is clearest and then refocusing the camera if necessary. If no improvement is noted, then the blurry view cannot be corrected with this device. In that case, set the knob back to the zero position and focus as best you can.

Although the astigmatism corrector is valuable for reducing the induced type of astigmatism introduced in peripheral

![Center for Sight eagle logo]

CENTER FOR SIGHT
GEORGETOWN UNIVERSITY MEDICAL CENTER

Posterior Segment Photography

Date: _____

Name: _____ DOB: _____ Age: _____ Sex: _____

Physician: _____ Referring Physician: _____

Address: _____

Ocular
Diagnosis: _____ ICD.9 Code(s) _____

Reason for Photos: _____

Visual Acuity		Media Opacity		Systemic Disease

Visual Acuity

OD _____

OS

Media Opacity

Cornea ☐ OD ☐ OS

Lens ☐ OD ☐ OS

Vitreous ☐ OD ☐ OS

Systemic Disease

☐ Diabetes

☐ Hypertension

☐ Other _____

IOP

OD _____

OS

Aphakic ☐ OD ☐ OS

Pseudophakic ☐ OD ☐ OS

Allergies

☐ Penicillin

☐ Other _____

Color Fundus Photography:

Eye(s)
☐ OD
☐ OS
☐ OU

Field(s)
☐ #1   Disc
☐ #2   Macula
☐ #1½   Disc & Macula
☐ #1-7 Diabetic Series
☐ Other _____

Drug Therapy

☐ Insulin

☐ INH

☐ Chloroquine

☐ Epinephrine

☐ Anticoagulant

☐ Other _____

OD   OS   Special Instructions:

( )   ( )

Stat Process: yes   no

Fluorescein Angiography:

Eye(s)
☐ OD
☐ OS
☐ OD/OS
☐ OS/OD

Transit Field
☐ #1   Disc
☐ #2   Macula
☐ #1½   Disc & Macula
☐ Other _____

FORM 5-1. A photographic requisition form for fundus photography and fluorescein angiography.

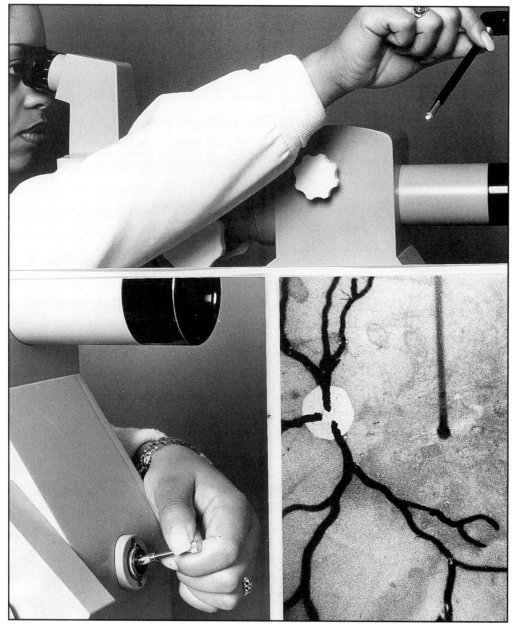

Figure 5-3. Devices for the patient to look at. Top: A fixation light can be used with patients who see with both eyes. Bottom left: An internal pointer or stick may be helpful for the monocular patient to fixate on. Bottom right: Unfortunately, this pointer is photographed along with the fundus (model eye).

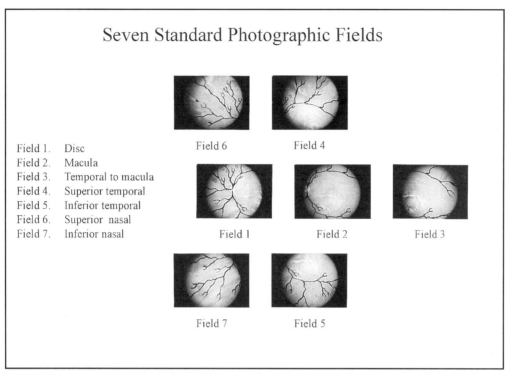

Seven Standard Photographic Fields

Field 1.   Disc
Field 2.   Macula
Field 3.   Temporal to macula
Field 4.   Superior temporal
Field 5.   Inferior temporal
Field 6.   Superior nasal
Field 7.   Inferior nasal

Field 6   Field 4

Field 1   Field 2   Field 3

Field 7   Field 5

Figure 5-4. The Seven Standard Photographic Fields encompass overlapping views of the left fundus (model eye).

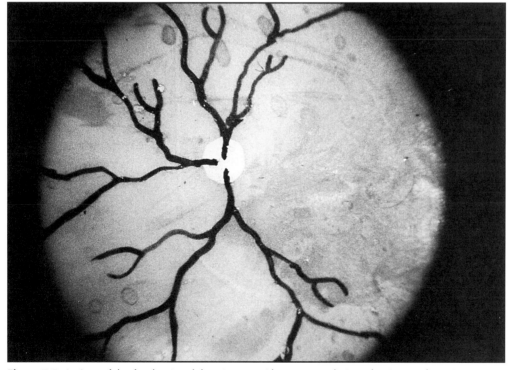

Figure 5-5. A view of the fundus (model eye) seen with a camera designed to image the retina at 30°.

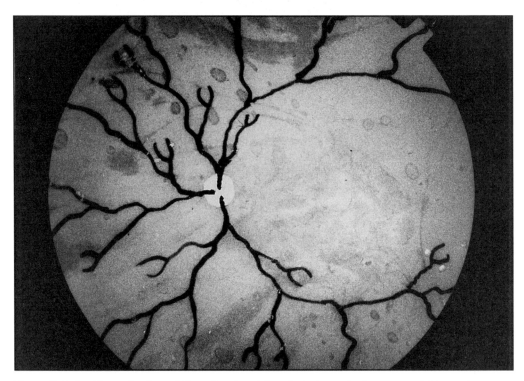

Figure 5-6. A wide-angle view of the retina (model eye) photographed with a variable angle camera set at 50°.

fundus photography, it can also be used on a patient with a refractive astigmatism. The procedure is the same as previously outlined.

Equipment

Although the fundus camera resembles a cannon, it is modeled after an indirect ophthalmoscope (Figure 5-8). It has, however, proven itself a useful weapon in the fight against visual loss by providing valuable information for the diagnosis and treatment of retinal disease.

A fundus camera consists of a main camera unit, base assembly, and power supply. The main unit is composed of an optical head, which houses an aspheric front lens and rear objective lens system, a flash bulb and viewing lamp, filters, mirrors, and on some cameras, an eyepiece assembly (Figure 5-9). A 35-mm SLR camera body is attached, although another kind of image-gathering device (such as an instant still or video camera) may be installed instead. The body of the 35-mm SLR functions primarily to hold and transport the film since it is used without a lens and does not play a role in image formation. When the camera is positioned properly, the pupil of the observer is aligned with the pupil of the patient for a magnified view of the retina.

The main camera unit is attached to a base that provides for patient positioning and camera movement. A power supply may be incorporated into the camera's base or stand alone, depending on its size. Controls for the viewing light, fixation light, and flash intensity, as well as the timer for fluorescein angiography, are often located on the face of the power source.

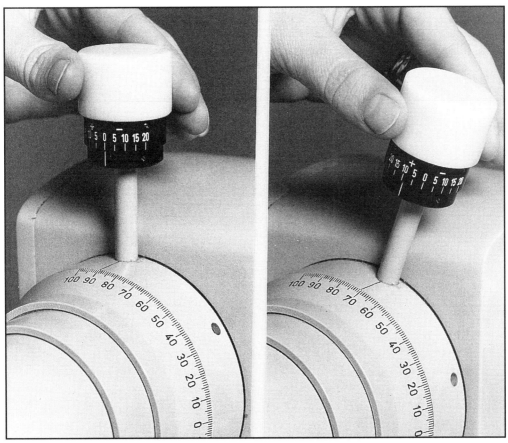

Figure 5-7. Using the astigmatism corrector featured on the Zeiss fundus camera.

Film

For ordinary documentation of intraocular conditions, daylight color positive transparency (slide) film is chosen for fundus photography. since the white light of the flash tube is balanced for use with this film. In general, a medium speed film (ISO 64-100) is utilized, although slower film may be used if the flash unit is powerful enough.

As previously mentioned, B&W fundus photography is effective in imaging the choroid, retinal vasculature, and nerve fiber layer when used with monochromatic illumination. If fluorescein angiography is to be performed along with monochromatic fundus photography, high speed B&W film (ISO 400) will provide acceptable results. If angiography is not being performed, however, consider using a slower speed film (ISO 100) to maximize the image definition.

Getting Ready

Before the Patient is Present

Whenever possible, the photographer should verify that the fundus camera is in working order before the patient enters the room. This equipment check is best done behind the scenes, espe-

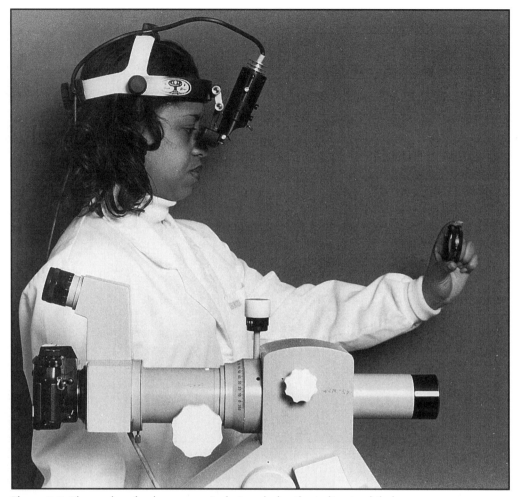

Figure 5-8. The modern fundus camera is designed after the indirect ophthalmoscope.

cially if the photographer is not particularly adept at camera maintenance. Witnessing an otherwise capable photographer fumble about trying to change a fuse or plug may be detrimental if the patient's confidence in the photographer's ability is shaken.

During this pre-patient check, make sure that the power unit is plugged in, all cords and cables are connected, the viewing lamp is lit, and the flash is firing. The designated 35-mm camera body should then be mounted to the fundus camera (Figure 5-10) and loaded with the appropriate film. If there is film in the camera, make sure that it is advancing properly. Be sure that the mounted camera's shutter speed is in synch with the flash of the fundus camera, and set the flash intensity to correspond with the speed of the film selected. If B&W monochromatic photography is being performed instead of color, make sure that the correct filter is in place.

After the Patient is Present

While introducing yourself to patients, size them up, observing their height, girth, and degree of pupillary dilation. Set the table to the appropriate height, then clean the face rest and adjust accordingly as you explain the procedure. If the patient's pupils are not well dilated, check to see if they need more drops or if you need to allow more time for the dilation to take effect. Inadequately dilated pupils are a major cause of poor quality fundus photography.

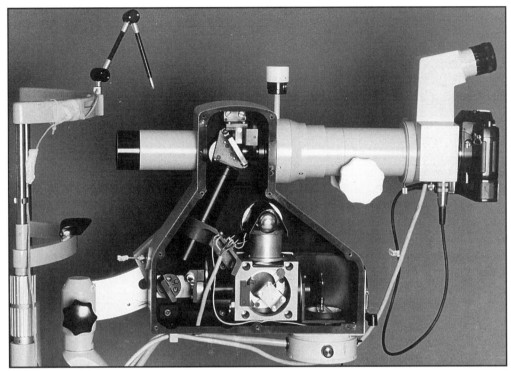

Figure 5-9. The inside of a working fundus camera.

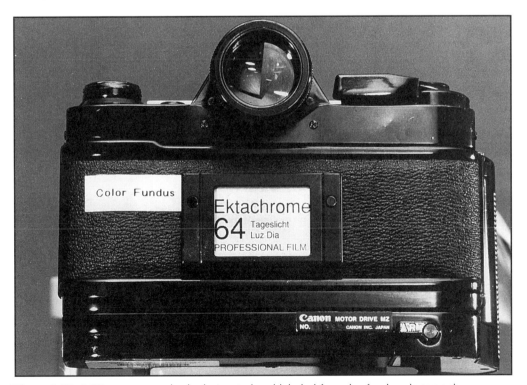

Figure 5-10. A 35-mm camera body designated and labeled for color fundus photography.

After reviewing the physician's orders, talk with the patient about the procedure, answering any questions he or she may have about the picture-taking session. Medical questions, of course, should be directed to the physician. Speak in a calm and reassuring tone. The voice of competence can inspire confidence. When the patient trusts the photographer as a capable professional, he or she is in a better position to cooperate. It is much easier to photograph a willing participant than a reluctant subject.

What the Patient Needs to Know

·   You are not being x-rayed.

·   Your pictures are being taken with ordinary color (or B&W) film.

·   The flash is bright, but it lasts only a fraction of a second.

·   Please follow the fixation light (or stick) with your eyes only.

·   Keep your head in the face rest so that you stay in the camera's focus range.

·   You may blink unless I say otherwise.

After you've explained what you'll be doing, wash your hands. (Do this in front of the patient.)

OptT Although it is customary to start with the right eye when checking visual acuity or tonometry, the order in which the eyes are imaged matters little in fundus photography. After the patient has come forward and placed his or her head in the face rest, position the camera at its recommended working distance in front of the eye to be photographed first. For most table-mounted fundus cameras, this camera-to-patient distance will be around 45 mm (measured from the camera's front lens to the patient's cornea), but a portable camera may have a working distance as short as 7 mm.[2] The exact working distance of your camera will be listed under the "specifications" section of the owner's manual but can also be approximated by sharply imaging the camera's circle of light directly onto the patient's closed eyelid (Figure 5-11). If you look at the patient's lid from alongside the camera, not through the ocular, this lighted circle is seen in clear focus when you are at the appropriate working distance.

With the patient's eye opened, you can confirm that you are at the correct working distance by looking into the eyepiece. When you are in proper range, the retina will be evenly illuminated. If you are too far from or too close to the eye, unwanted light reflections will appear in the picture instead.

OptT If you are off center, a crescent-shaped light reflection will be seen (Figure 5-12) since a portion of the circular illumination light, or "donut," is bouncing off the iris rather than the retina. To get rid of this crescent, move the camera's joystick in the direction opposite the unwanted reflection. If your patient is not adequately dilated, it may be impossible to eliminate this artifact entirely.

Once the donut of light is properly aligned, you are almost ready to take a picture, but don't trip the shutter quite yet. Bring your attention to the grid inside the eyepiece. This grid (aka, cross hairs, reticle, or reticule), superimposed over the magnified view of your patient's retina, is quite easy to overlook or ignore, but its focus is crucial if clear pictures are desired. You may encounter any one of four possible situations (Figure 5-13) when you look through the eyepiece of the fun-

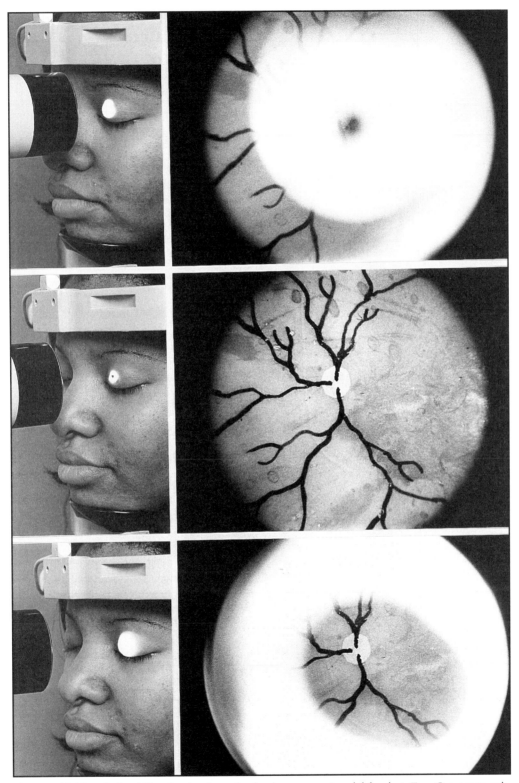

Figure 5-11. The circle of illumination from the fundus camera (model fundus). Top: Camera-to-subject distance is too close. Middle: Camera-to-subject distance is just right. Bottom: Camera-to-subject distance is too far away.

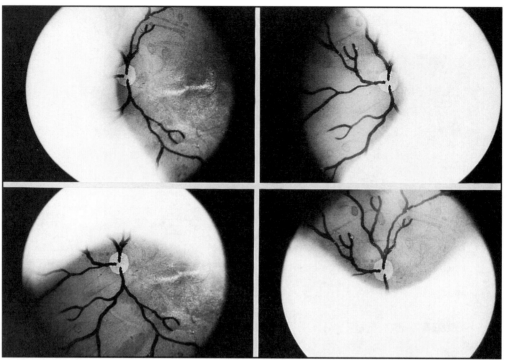

Figure 5-12. When the camera is not centered properly, crescent-shaped artifacts of illumination appear (model eye).

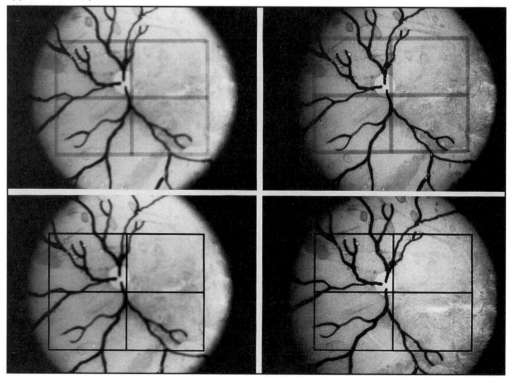

Figure 5-13. A photographer's view of the retina (model eye) through the camera's eyepiece. Top left: Retina and reticle are both out of focus. Top right: Retina is in focus, but the reticle is out of focus. Bottom left: Retina is out of focus, but the reticle is in focus. Bottom right: Retina and reticle are both in focus.

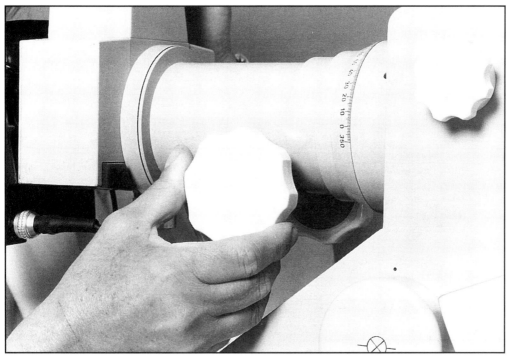

Figure 5-14. This knob is used to focus the patient's retina.

dus camera, but only the combination of both a focused grid and sharp retinal image will result in a good picture.

Getting the retina in sharp focus is easy. Just turn the appropriate knob (Figure 5-14) until you get a clear view. However, even when the retina is sharply seen through the eyepiece, if the grid is blurry, an out-of-focus photograph will result. Only a focused grid will insure that the camera is seeing exactly what you, the photographer, are seeing. In other words, focusing the grid compensates for your refractive error.

To set the grid, first focus on your patient's retina using your distance vision. At the same time, and while continuing to look at the retina, notice whether the grid is sharp or blurry. (Do not shift your focus from the retina to the grid or you will accommodate). Try to maintain only a visual awareness of the grid. Still without looking directly at the grid, turn the knob of the eyepiece all the way to the "plus" indicator (Figure 5-15, left). Then, slowly turn the knob toward the "minus" side until the grid appears sharp (See Figure 5-15, right). Stop. Do not go beyond this point or you will stimulate accommodation, and you will have to start all over again. When both the grid and the retina are clearly focused, you may take a picture.

Because of their tremendous ability to accommodate, young photographers may find that setting the grid properly is difficult and may be their biggest hurdle in taking sharp pictures. Patience and persistence will help the "youngsters" master the art of setting the grid, but only the loss of accommodation (aging) will make it effortless.

Stereoscopic Fundus Photography

For a picture to appear more realistic, in addition to demonstrating the height and width of a subject, depth must also be conveyed. Depth, the third dimension (3-D), exists in reality but can

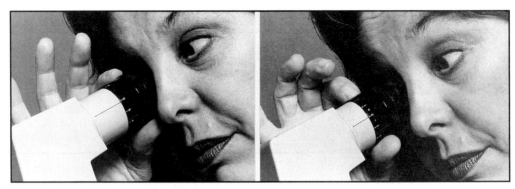

Figure 5-15. Focusing the reticle. Left: First, turn the eyepiece all the way to the plus (+) side. Right: Then, while looking through the viewfinder, turn the eyepiece toward the minus (-) side. Once the grid appears sharp, STOP or you may stimulate accommodation making it necessary to begin the process again.

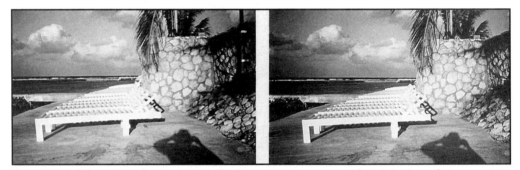

Figure 5-16. When viewed stereoscopically, these two pictures provide a 3-D view of Montego Bay, Jamaica. They were taken simultaneously using two identical 35-mm cameras spaced approximately 100 mm apart. For a stereo view, use your left eye to look at the left print and your right eye to view the right print. This method of viewing may be done with or without magnification.

also be recreated if a subject is photographed stereoscopically.

In the 1850s, after great success in Europe, stereo photography was introduced in the United States where it flourished. Viewing a 3-D stereograph of far away places allowed millions of Americans to see the world without leaving home. Today, stereo photographs are still used to entertain (Figure 5-16), but in the medical field, they are used to evaluate patients and educate health care professionals. In eyecare, the ubiquitous fly test—a simple yet effective tool for evaluating a patient's stereoscopic depth perception—is one way in which stereo techniques are applied during an eye examination. Taking stereo pictures of the ocular fundus is another.

Those of us with stereoscopic vision perceive depth because our brains are capable of combining the two slightly different views provided by each eye into one picture. During stereo fundus photography, we use a single fundus camera to take two pictures of the same subject, also from a slightly different position, mimicking the view seen with each eye. Although both pictures of the fundus may be taken simultaneously with a special stereo camera, most stereo photographs are taken in sequence using an ordinary fundus camera, and the resultant slides are generally viewed with magnification from a pair of plus (+) lenses with illumination from a light box.

With a well-dilated eye, the technique is simple. First, center the illumination donut on the patient's pupil with the joystick vertically oriented, and take the first picture. Move the camera at least 1 mm (about the width of a dime) laterally to the left or right, and take the second picture

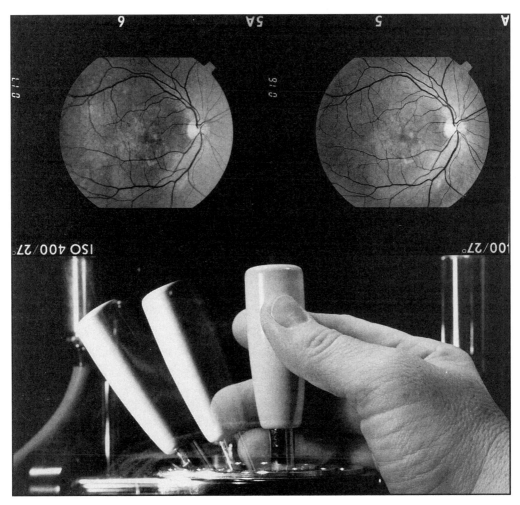

Figure 5-17. Performing stereoscopic fundus photography. Top: When these two monochromatic fundus photographs are viewed in stereo, the brain "sees" a single image of an elevated choroidal lesion. (Although the film's frame numbers and ISO designation are upside down, the film is properly oriented for viewing as this is a right eye.) Bottom: To obtain the above "stereo pair," the first picture (frame #5) was taken with the joystick oriented vertically and the camera's illumination light centered on the pupil, aimed at the macula. Then the joystick was moved a little bit to the left and a second picture (frame #6) was taken of the same subject from a slightly different position. Note: If the resultant slides (or pictures) are mounted (or printed) individually, the second half of the stereo pair may be taken with the joystick moved to *either* the left or right of its original position. When the end product is a negative strip or contact print, however, the joystick must be moved to the left for proper stereo viewing.

(Figure 5-17). A good 3-D representation of the subject will result if the eye remains stationary. Patients with small pupils and roving eyes make stereo fundus photography more difficult.

Problems and Solutions

Establishing the appropriate working distance and carefully aligning the fundus camera is the first step toward obtaining pictures of the inner eye. Getting both the retina and the eyepiece grid

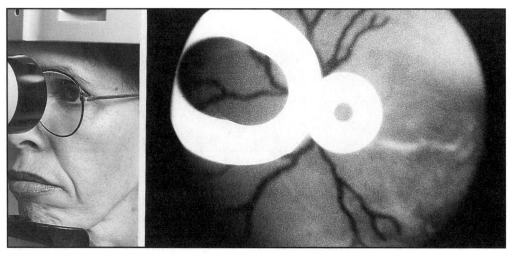

Figure 5-18. When a patient is photographed with her spectacles on, an interesting artifact appears (model fundus).

in clear focus will help insure that these images are sharp. Even with good preliminary camera technique, photographing a living subject can still prove to be quite challenging. The patients themselves can introduce all sorts of interesting problems to the photographic session.

When your patient is emmetropic or has only a small refractive error, the standard lens on the fundus camera is used. Patients with refractive errors greater than the range covered by the camera's standard lens need to be optically corrected if sharp fundus photographs are to be obtained. If your patient wears contact lenses, the necessary correction may be obtained by photographing the eye with the contact in place using the standard camera lens. Spectacles, however, may not be worn during fundus photography since unwanted reflections will be introduced by the glasses (Figure 5-18). The patient's optical correction must then be provided by the fundus camera.

Before you have the patient remove his or her glasses, decide whether the lenses have plus (+) or minus (-) power. Plus lenses will magnify the wearer's eyes, while minus lenses will make the eyes look smaller. Then, based on your observation, dial in either a plus or minus lens using the camera's diopter compensation device (Figure 5-19). Have the patient remove the glasses, then proceed with fundus photography.

Dialing in the plus lens on the diopter compensation device will also enable you to take external eye photographs with the fundus camera. Even though a fundus camera is designed to be used on the concave surface of the inner eye, it will often provide satisfactory (though not optimal) results when used on the convex surface of the outer eye (Figure 5-20).

A droopy upper eyelid needs to be lifted or the retina won't be evenly illuminated. Although the shape of this artifact is quite similar to the pattern seen on the visual field of a patient with ptosis (Figure 5-21), it will be seen in the bottom of the photograph rather than the top. This occurs because the lid is outside the working distance of the fundus camera. Likewise, a single upper eyelash that is in the way will show up on the lower portion of the fundus photo (Figure 5-22).

A media opacity such as a cataract may make it difficult to get a good look at the ocular fundus, but sometimes this view can be improved if a clearer port of entry into the eye is found (Figure 5-23). Careful manipulation of the joystick is the easiest way to dodge such media opacities while searching for a better view.

Camera malfunctions and problems can occur intermittently or even when the equipment

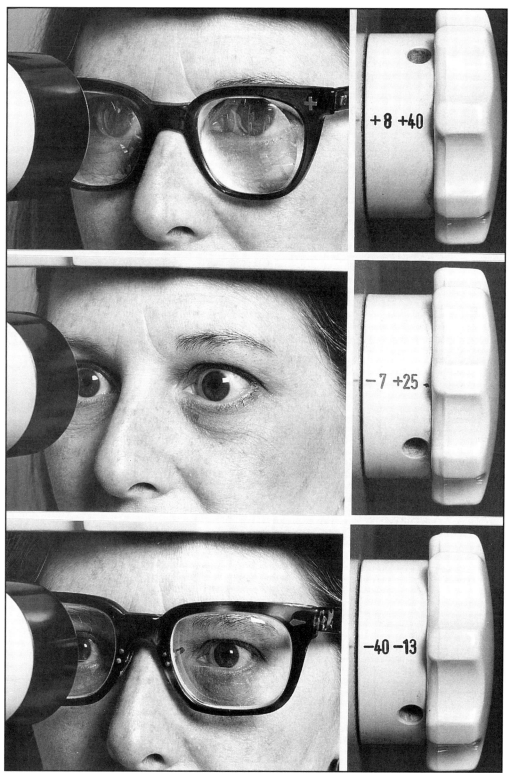

Figure 5-19. If your patient's correction is outside the normal limits of your fundus camera, dial in a extra plus (+) or minus (-) power with the appropriate knobs. (The patient's glasses were left on for demonstration purposes.)

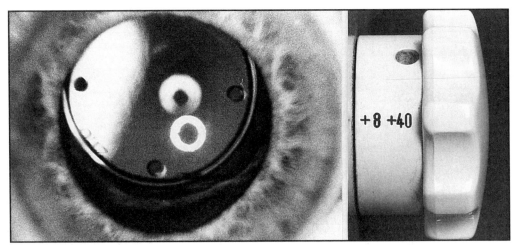

Figure 5-20. Adjusting the diopter compensation device to a high plus setting allows the front of the eye to be photographed with a fundus camera. Left: An external view of an eye with an intraocular lens photographed with a fundus camera. Right: The plus knob in position.

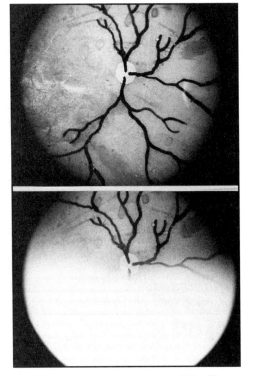
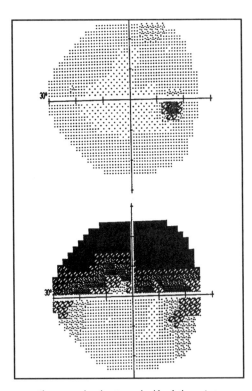

Figure 5-21. A droopy upper eyelid will appear as an artifact on the bottom half of the picture—exactly opposite from where it would be seen on a visual field of the same eye (model eye). Top row: An eye with the lids wide apart. Bottom row: A droopy top lid seen as an artifact in the fundus photograph and visual field (Visual fields performed by Elizabeth Aiken Burt, COT).

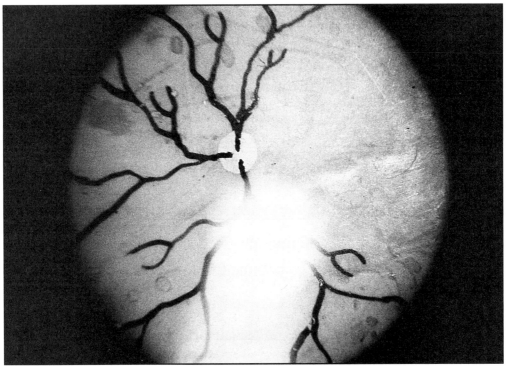

Figure 5-22. A single eyelash from above will be seen below, producing a white artifact at the bottom of the photo.

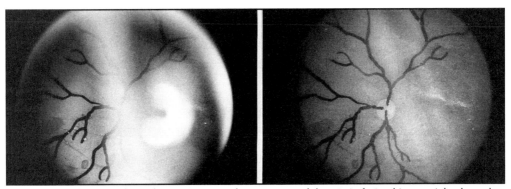

Figure 5-23. The view through a cataract is often poor (model eye). Left: Looking straight through the opacity. Right: The same eye photographed through a clearer portion of the lens. Although the view is low in contrast, it is adequate for assessing the retina.

seems to be operating well (Figure 5-24). If you have your film developed promptly, you can get photographic evidence of malfunctions before rolls and rolls of film have been wasted. If you suspect that a camera is broken, take it out of circulation immediately and have it repaired. This can save both you and the patient the time and expense of retaking the photographs.

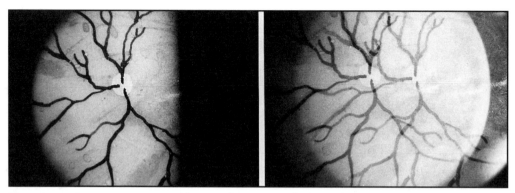

Figure 5-24. Common camera problems. Left: Improper flash synchronization. This picture was taken with the shutter set at 1/125th of a second instead of 1/60th of a second. Right: A double exposure.

Conclusion

Although many practitioners still use colored pencils to sketch out their findings on a piece of paper, photography is more accurate and has largely supplanted drawing. Careful attention to camera technique coupled with consideration for the patient will assure that this accuracy is not obtained at the expense of the patient's comfort.

References

1. Diabetic Retinopathy Study Research Group. Report 7. A modification of the Airlie House classification of diabetic retinopathy. *Invest Ophthalmol Vis Sci.* 1981;21(1):212.
2. Cunningham D. Establishing the working distance in fundus photography. *Viewpoints (Journal of the Association of Technical Personnel in Ophthalmology).* 1991; 7.

Chapter 6

Fluorescein Angiography

KEY POINTS

- Use a requisition form to eliminate confusion by enhancing communication.

- Advocate and document informed consent.

- Have an emergency medical kit readily available, and inspect its contents on a regular schedule.

- Perform color photography first.

- The filling stages of a fluorescein angiogram are the choroidal flush, followed by the arterial, early venous, full venous, and late phases.

Purpose

If color fundus photography is a good way to show what structures look like inside the eye, then fluorescein angiography is best at demonstrating how these structures work. Although developed initially as a research tool, over time fluorescein angiography has established itself in the clinical arena as a means of evaluating the cause of unexplained decreased visual acuity. It is highly regarded by those who diagnose and treat diseases and disorders of the ocular fundus.

Indications

Because fluorescein dye does not normally leak from the blood vessels inside the eye, fluorescein angiography has proven to be a useful diagnostic aid in the understanding of retinal vascular disease. Abnormalities in flow characteristics and circulation times can be recorded with this technique. If a retinal artery, vein, or capillary is blocked, the site of the occlusion can be pinpointed and the damage to the surrounding tissue assessed. In addition, when blood vessels are leaking, the abnormal structures and resultant seepage of blood products can be identified by their visible fluorescence. In cases where laser intervention is necessary, a good quality angiogram provides the ophthalmologist with a map for the treatment session.

Fluorescein angiography is considered essential in the management of many vision-threatening conditions that affect the macula. In the severe form of age-related macular degeneration (the leading cause of visual loss among the older population), blood vessels from the choroid may grow under the retina and leak fluid or bleed. A fluorescein angiogram can identify these unwanted vessels and provide a guide for laser therapy.

Problems that affect the macula may have their origin elsewhere in the eye or body. Although visual symptoms, such as blurring or distortion, may be explained by an accumulation of fluid in the macula, the source of the leak may be far removed from the symptomatic area. Choroidal melanomas, optic nerve pits, and other ocular lesions located outside the macular region have been diagnosed after being discovered during fluorescein angiography for macular edema.

It is not uncommon for disorders and diseases of other organs of the body to be accompanied or followed by manifestations of eye disease. Diabetes mellitus destroys capillaries, so most diabetic patients will develop abnormalities of their retinal blood vessels. Fluorescein angiography is an extremely valuable test for patients with diabetic retinopathy.

Physician's Orders

To maximize the informational content of a fluorescein angiogram, the study should be individually tailored to the patient's problem and the physician's expectations. As ocular photographers, we are responsible for gathering this critical information, and it is helpful to do this before the patient is seated in front of the fundus camera. We should be able to answer the following questions—the Five W's of fluorescein angiography. Who is our patient, what is to be photographed, and where can it be found? Being told that Jane Doe has a hemorrhage in her right macula is a good start. Knowing when the problem is best demonstrated during the angiogram and why the study was ordered is equally important if your goal is to provide the most information possible. For example, being told ahead of time that recording the arterial phase is crucial to rule out a subretinal neovascular membrane is a great help for planning the photographic session.

For best results, ask these questions before the dye has been injected into the patient's blood stream. The answers are invaluable. Verbal orders are acceptable if your physician communicates his or her wishes clearly, but the use of a written requisition form (FORM 6-1) may eliminate confusion and will help to insure that the study is "just what the doctor ordered."

The Angiogram

The Monochromatic Photograph

Fluorescein angiography does not replace the clinical examination, it merely augments it. In situations where the interpreting physician has not personally examined the patient, however, color fundus photographs may serve as a suitable stand-in. Sometimes neither the patient nor the color photographs are available for comparison. Taking a picture of the affected eye(s) at the beginning of every B&W roll of film used for angiography (before the exciter and barrier filters are in place and the dye has been injected) provides an ophthalmoscopic representation for inspection (Figure 6-1, top left/no time). On most cameras, a green filter is provided for taking this monochromatic (or "red-free") photograph since green light enhances the visibility of the retinal blood vessels.

The Control Photograph

When a "control" photograph of a patient's inner eye is taken with the exciter and barrier filters in place before the injection of fluorescein dye, the resultant image should appear totally dark (See Figure 6-1, 000.0 sec). This pre-injection photograph is an important part of every angiographic study for checking the integrity of the filters in use. If an image of the patient's fundus can be seen in this frame, the filters may need to be replaced.

Phases of the Normal Angiogram

In general, the initial filling of fluorescein dye (the transit) is recorded along with additional views taken approximately 10 minutes after, during the late phase. If you are not exactly sure when to document what, ask your doctor. Learn the names of the circulation phases of fluorescein to enhance communication with referring physicians and become familiar with the normal route and characteristic appearance of the dye inside the eye. This way, the dye's movement can be anticipated and captured photographically, despite its transient nature.

On average, it takes from 10 to 15 seconds for a rapid injection of dye to travel from the vein in the arm to the ophthalmic artery, which then delivers the fluorescein to the eye. This is called the arm-to-retina circulation time. If your patient is shorter or taller than average or the injection is faster or slower than usual, the dye may be seen sooner or later than expected.

The first part of the transit of a fluorescein angiogram is called the choroidal flush or phase. As fluorescein dye enters the eye, a faint and patchy glow may be seen in the choroid. The overlying retinal vessels remain dark and are visible only in silhouette. This phase is best seen in lightly pigmented fundi (Figure 6-2). In darker eyes, it may not be possible to record the choroidal flush as an isolated event because the pigmented layer of the retina can mask out this weak burst of initial fluorescence. If a cilioretinal artery is present, it will light up during this phase of the angiogram.

CENTER FOR SIGHT

GEORGETOWN UNIVERSITY MEDICAL CENTER

Posterior Segment Photography

Date: _____

Name: _____ DOB: _____ Age: _____ Sex: _____

Physician: _____ Referring Physician: _____

Address: _____

Ocular
Diagnosis: _____ ICD.9 Code(s) _____

Reason for Photos: _____

Visual Acuity		Media Opacity			Systemic Disease	
OD	_____	Cornea	☐ OD	☐ OS	☐ Diabetes	
OS		Lens	☐ OD	☐ OS	☐ Hypertension	
		Vitreous	☐ OD	☐ OS	☐ Other _____	
IOP					**Allergies**	
OD	_____	Aphakic	☐ OD	☐ OS		
OS		Pseudophakic	☐ OD	☐ OS	☐ Penicillin	
					☐ Other _____	

Drug Therapy

Color Fundus Photography:

Eye(s)
- ☐ OD
- ☐ OS
- ☐ OU

Field(s)
- ☐ #1   Disc
- ☐ #2   Macula
- ☐ #1½ Disc & Macula
- ☐ #1-7 Diabetic Series
- ☐ Other _____

Drug Therapy
- ☐ Insulin
- ☐ INH
- ☐ Chloroquine
- ☐ Epinephrine
- ☐ Anticoagulant
- ☐ Other _____

OD   OS

Special Instructions:

Stat Process: yes   no

Fluorescein Angiography:

Eye(s)
- ☐ OD
- ☐ OS
- ☐ OD/OS
- ☐ OS/OD

Transit Field
- ☐ #1   Disc
- ☐ #2   Macula
- ☐ #1½ Disc & Macula
- ☐ Other _____

FORM 6-1. Photographic requisition to be used for fluorescein angiography and/or fundus photography.

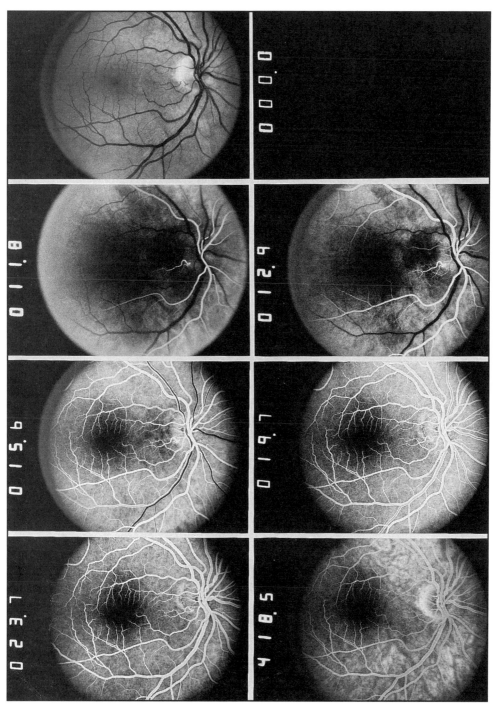

Figure 6-1. Select frames from a normal fluorescein angiogram. Top left: No time monochromatic. Top right: 000.0-sec control. Second row left: 011.8-sec arterial phase. Second row right: 012.9-sec very early venous phase. Third row left: 015.6-sec early venous (laminar flow) phase. Third row right: 019.7-sec laminar flow continued. Bottom left: 023.7-sec full venous phase. Bottom right: 418.5-sec late phase.

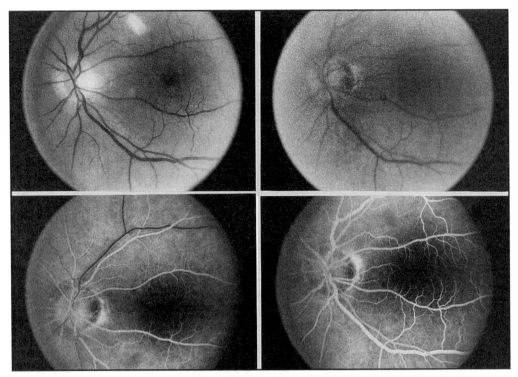

Figure 6-2. A fluorescein angiogram of the left eye of a patient with an obvious choroidal flush. Top left: Monochromatic. Top right: Choroidal flush. Bottom left: Venous laminar flow. Bottom right: Late phase.

Next, the central retinal artery fills and all the retinal arterioles fluoresce very quickly during what is called the arterial phase (See Figure 6-1, 011.8 sec). At this point, the dye is flowing away from the optic nerve. After working its way through the capillary bed, the dye changes direction and flows back toward the optic nerve through the venules and veins. During the early venous phase, fluorescence is seen only along the outside edges of the veins. This striped pattern is called laminar flow because of the layered appearance of the dye (See Figure 6-1, 012.9 sec).

Venous filling is slower than arterial filling, so this pattern of fluorescence can continue for a few seconds (See Figure 6-1, 015.6 sec and 019.7 sec). When fluorescein has mixed with all the blood inside the veins, the full venous phase is in progress (See Figure 6-1, 023.7 sec). At this time, all the arteries, capillaries, and veins inside the eye will glow, making it difficult to distinguish a vein from an artery based on its fluorescent appearance alone.

As time passes, the retinal vessels empty of the fluorescein-dyed blood. During this late phase of the angiogram, only a small amount of background fluorescence from the choroid will be seen along with staining around the optic nerve (See Figure 6-1, 418.5 sec).

Throughout the fluorescein angiogram of a normal eye, the macula will remain dark because of the increased pigmentation in the cells of the retinal pigment epithelium. In addition, the presence of a yellow pigment (xanthophyll) in the macular region absorbs some of the blue exciting light. Another factor is that the center of the macula has no blood vessels. Since fluorescein dye moves through the eye with the blood, lack of blood vessels means lack of normal fluorescence in this area (Figure 6-3).

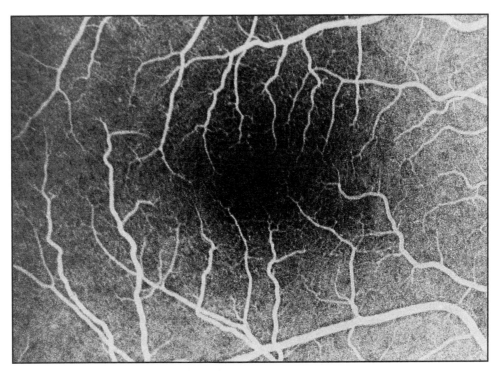

Figure 6-3. A frame from a fluorescein angiogram enlarged to show the avascular macula.

Principles of Fluorescence

Light is a form of radiant energy that can be seen by the human eye. It is a part of the electromagnetic spectrum, which is divided into several frequency bands extending from the extremely high frequency of gamma rays to the very low frequency of the microwaves of radar, television, and short-wave radio. Visible light consists of frequencies producing different color sensations and is usually defined by wavelength. Because wavelength is small, it is measured in metric units called nanometers (nm). One nanometer is equal to one-billionth of a meter or 1×10^{-9} m. This is indeed small when you consider that the diameter of a human hair is about 60 000 nm.

In order to become proficient as an angiographer, the normal flow characteristics of fluorescein sodium and how it looks inside the eye must be learned (preceding section). The principles of fluorescence explain how and why we are able to produce such an awesome effect.

Fluorescence is a form of light. A primary source of light, like the sun or an ordinary light bulb (Figure 6-4), emits light produced by heat. This is called incandescence. Objects are made visible by reflecting and/or absorbing the light originating from this source. Emission of light due to causes other than intense heat is called luminescence. During luminescence, incidental light energy causes the electrons of the atoms of the absorbing material to become excited and jump from the inner orbits of the atoms to the outer orbits. When the electrons fall back to their original state, a photon of light is emitted and the material glows. If the glow continues for an appreciable time after the exciting light has been removed (Figure 6-5), this is termed phosphorescence. If the glow stops shortly after the exciting light has been taken away (Figure 6-6), this is called fluorescence.

In a darkened examination room, you may notice that your watch dial glows. You are wit-

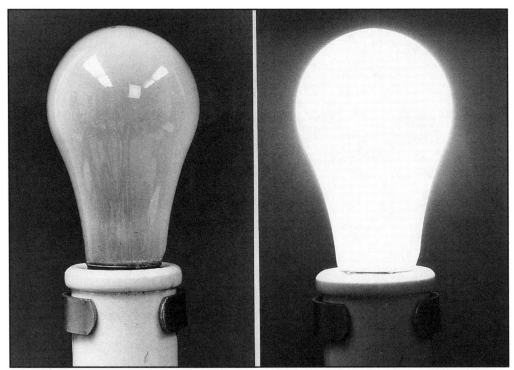

Figure 6-4. An ordinary incandescent light bulb. Left: Turned off. Right: Turned on and glowing.

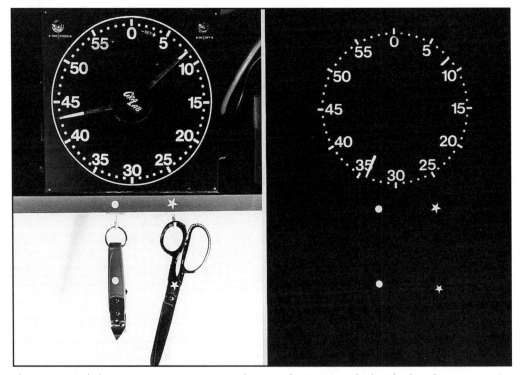

Figure 6-5. A darkroom timer, can opener, and a pair of scissors marked with phosphorescent paint or stickers. Left: The room lights are on. Right: The room lights are off and the phosphorescent numbers and stickers are glowing.

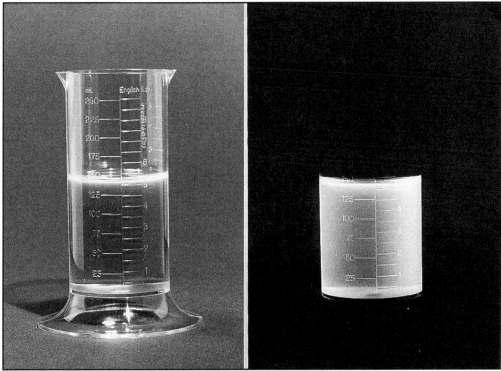

Figure 6-6. A graduated cylinder filled with flourescein dye and water. Left: The room lights are on. Right: The room lights are off, and a blue exciter light causes the liquid to glow. A barrier filter was also employed to allow only fluorescent light to be recorded on film.

nessing the phosphorescent form of luminescence. When you stain a corneal abrasion with fluorescein, you will see that it glows too, but only for as long as the blue light is directed at the subject. This is the fluorescent form of luminescence. Because fluorescence does not linger, you will not see an afterglow when you take the light away.

In the ophthalmic setting, intravenous fluorescein angiography is the most dramatic application of fluorescence. When fluorescein dye has blended with the blood inside the retinal vessels, the resultant mixture is a potential source of light rather than the object of reflected light. With proper stimulation, the fluoresceinated blood will glow.

Materials that fluoresce will glow when excited by light of a specific color or wavelength. The fluorescein dye used in ophthalmology absorbs blue light at a wavelength between 465 nm and 490 nm and emits a yellowish green light at 520 nm to 530 nm. Although the excited fluorescein molecules have stepped up to a longer wavelength and higher frequency, the glow is of a lesser energy level (Figure 6-7). During fluorescein angiography, we capture this phenomenon photographically.

Filters Used in Fluorescein Angiography

Exciter Filter

The photographic techniques used during fluorescein angiography are similar to those employed in routine fundus photography, but the color of the illumination source is noticeably

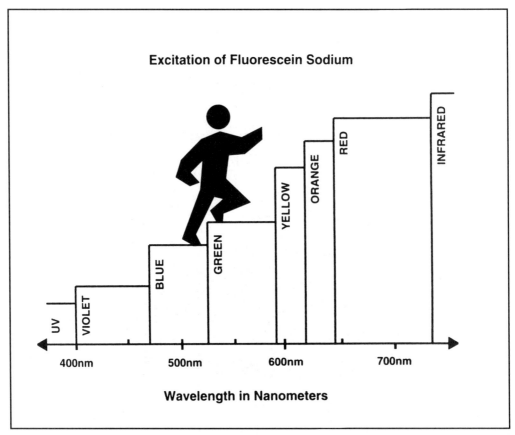

Figure 6-7. A graphic representation of what happens when a molecule of fluorescein dye is exposed to the blue light. After it absorbs the blue light (465-490 nm), it "steps up" to a higher wavelength (520-530 nm) and emits a yellowish-green light.

different. Only blue light of the proper wavelength can be used to stimulate fluorescein dye, so a blue filter is placed inside the fundus camera in the path of the light. This filter transmits only radiation, which excites the molecules of dye and (in theory) absorbs all other wavelengths. If retinal blood vessels contain fluorescein dye, they will glow when the blue light from this exciter filter is aimed at them.

Barrier Filter

Once excited by the blue light of the flash, the dye will emit a yellow-green glow. Even though our eyes can distinguish between the blue reflected light and the yellowish fluorescent glow, the film is not nearly as sensitive to such subtle differences in color. In order to accentuate the all-important fluorescent light, the blue light must be eliminated before it hits the film. A yellow barrier filter placed in front of the film will serve to absorb this unwanted blue light.

Equipment

The fundus camera used during color photography can also be used for fluorescein angiography if it is equipped with the appropriate filters (exciter and barrier) and has a flash of sufficient power to excite the dye. In addition, the flash unit must recycle quickly in order to record the rapid movement of the dye. An internal device capable of marking each photographic frame with the elapsed time is useful as well and may prove to be invaluable if any abnormality in circulation is present.

It is necessary to use a fast B&W film (ISO 400) with most cameras to record the small amount of fluorescence emitted from the inner eye. If you are recording onto a computer chip rather than onto a piece of photographic film, your video camera must have the sensitivity to pick up the very low level of light available in fundus fluorescein angiography.

In addition to having the necessary equipment, it is essential that you are knowledgeable about the procedure and have had proper training. Gaining proficiency in the craft of fundus photography will best help you prepare for fluorescein angiography.

Preparation

For best results, the photographer must be skilled in both camera technique and patient management. High-quality equipment and an understanding of the way dye flows through the eye are important, but will not substitute for actual experience behind the fundus camera working with live patients. If you are routinely performing fundus photography, the transition to fluorescein angiography is usually not difficult since the camera movements and patient positions are the same. But if you have little or no experience with a fundus camera, do not attempt fluorescein angiography until you have acquired some hands-on training.

Your patients will also need some training if you expect them to actively participate in the process. Remember, without your patient's cooperation, a fluorescein angiogram is nearly impossible to obtain. Patient training can be easily incorporated into the color fundus photography session if it is done prior to fluorescein angiography. At this more relaxed pace, patients can learn and practice their role in front of the camera without a needle sticking in their arm. This time also gives you an opportunity to assess your patient's abilities. You may notice that he doesn't see the fixation light well, or that she closes her eyes and opens her mouth. These concerns can often be remedied through verbal encouragement or a change in technique and are best addressed during color fundus photography.

Color fundus photography is unsurpassed as a training tool for the patient and photographer about to embark on fluorescein angiography. If you are tempted to rush right into the angiogram, it may help to know that color fundus photographs taken after an injection of fluorescein may result in an inaccurate color representation of the ocular fundus.[1] For best results, take color fundus photos first.

Complications

As stated previously, only a proficient fundus photographer should perform fluorescein angiography. Once injected into the blood stream, fluorescein makes its passage through the retinal circulation so quickly that an unskilled photographer could easily miss its initial trip through the eye. Because the transit phase of the angiogram sometimes provides the most useful information, a study lacking these valuable photographs may prove to be inadequate for purposes of interpretation or treatment. In this case, the angiogram must be repeated and the patient subjected to an additional dose of the dye. Although animal studies have shown a lethal dose to be about 100 times the amount used clinically, in a fluorescein-sensitive patient even the recommended dose may result in an untoward reaction.[2]

The nature and severity of complications associated with fluorescein angiography can be categorized as mild, moderate, or severe. Nausea is the most common mild adverse reaction, with vomiting reported less frequently. The photographer's role is to comfort the patient and provide an emesis basin if necessary.

Moderate reactions to fluorescein dye include hives, shortness of breath, rash, and fever; these require some form of medical intervention. Because of this, a physician and crash cart should be available whenever and wherever angiography is performed. It is recommended that all photographers be aware of the expected and possible reactions to the dye, be able to recognize the signs of respiratory or cardiac arrest, and know how to perform cardiopulmonary resuscitation (CPR). (In fact, CPR training is considered essential and is required for certification for many eye care professions.) It is comforting to know that certified ophthalmic assistants, technicians, technologists, and photographers must be proficient in CPR since serious, life-threatening adverse reactions to the dye can occur, and fluorescein-related deaths have been reported.

A more common complication of fluorescein angiography occurs at the injection site when the needle is displaced and the dye escapes from the blood vessel into which it was injected, infiltrating the surrounding tissue. This extravasation of dye (Figure 6-8) can cause intense pain at the site or a dull, aching pain in the arm. Utilizing careful intravenous technique and verifying proper placement of the needle before pushing the dye will help avoid this unwelcome complication.

Informed Consent

A physician cannot perform a procedure on a patient without ensuring that the patient understands the purpose of the procedure and has been informed of its potential risks and benefits. An informed patient can make a knowledgeable decision to accept or reject the recommended procedure. The process of obtaining a patient's permission is called informed consent. If the patient is a minor (Figure 6-9) or has become incompetent through illness or injury, his or her parent(s) or guardian has the authority to consent to medical care.

What the Patient Needs to Know

- These pictures will be taken using ordinary colored light, not x-radiation or laser light.
- It takes approximately _____ minutes to complete this test.
- Your permission is required to do this test. You will be informed about the procedure before giving your written consent. Please ask questions about anything you do not understand.
- Although most patients tolerate this procedure well, a few experience brief nausea following the injection of dye. Since this passes quickly, try to remain at the camera. On rare occasions, someone may react to the dye by vomiting.
- Your urine and skin may be temporarily discolored because of the dye.
- For the results of your test, contact your doctor in approximately _____ hours/days.

Documenting informed consent (FORM 6-2) has become a routine part of fluorescein angiography in many practices. The actual consent form has legal importance, but the true value of

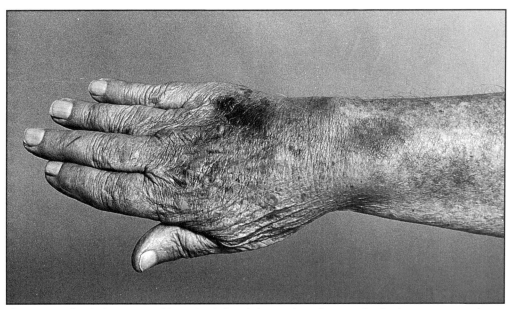

Figure 6-8. The dark areas on this patient's hand show where fluorescein dye has extravasated.

informed consent lies in the process of obtaining such consent. During this process, the risks and benefits of fluorescein angiography are discussed with explanations given and questions answered. When used appropriately, the potential benefits of fluorescein angiography have been judged to far outweigh the possible risks. It is the patient, however, not the doctor or the photographer, who must decide his or her tolerance of certain risks and give permission to proceed. In some cases, despite our best efforts at assuring them of the relative safety of the procedure, patients may refuse to be photographed. That is their right.

The Actual Angiogram

After the procedure has been explained to the patient and he or she has consented to proceed, the necessary supplies (Figure 6-10) and personnel must be gathered. These include a tourniquet, butterfly needle, vial of fluorescein dye, syringe, alcohol wipe, gauze pad, adhesive bandage, patient, and medical personnel to inject the dye. Because the public is keenly aware of disease transmission via shared needles, whenever possible, open the syringe and draw the dye in the presence of the patient so that he or she may see that the syringe is sterile and unused.

Perform color photography as usual, then prepare for angiography by loading the appropriate camera with B&W film (Figure 6-11). Shoot an ID tag of the patient's name, position the patient in front of the camera, and take monochromatic views of both eyes with the green filter. With the fluorescein filters in place, take a control photograph of the eye to be studied and set the timer to zero. After a suitable site has been found to inject the dye, the photographer should first signal the injector to push the fluorescein into the vein, then start the camera's timer. The transit of dye through the eye of primary interest is then photographed in rapid sequence, followed by representative views of the other eye. The needle can then be removed and, a short while later, late views of both eyes should be obtained. Then the film can be rewound, unloaded, and processed.

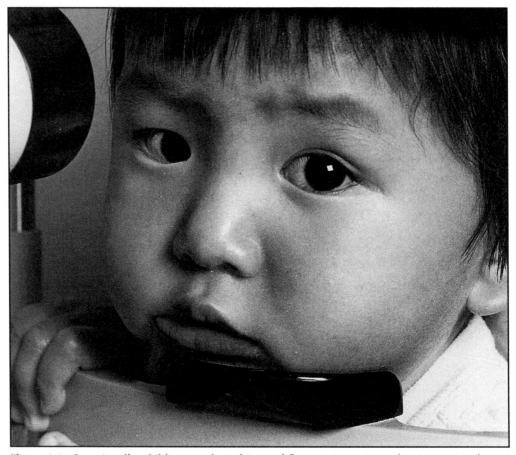

Figure 6-9. Occasionally, children are the subjects of fluorescein angiography. Permission from a parent or guardian is required before doing such an invasive procedure.

Processing and Presentation

Like all light-sensitive photographic materials, the B&W film used in fluorescein angiography must be chemically processed in order to make the latent image visible. To boost the inherently weak output and low contrast of the light emitted by fluorescence, a high-energy developer is needed. Because this is not a general-purpose developer, the data sheet included in the film box will not be helpful. In this case, follow the recommendation of the fundus camera's manufacturer or an experienced ophthalmic photographer with regard to selecting a developer and time, temperature, and agitation.

Once developed, the B&W roll of negative film is cut into short strips of five or six frames each and placed in a negative holder for protection. If your physician reads negatives, this will end your darkroom involvement.

Interpretation

Interpreting fluorescein angiograms is clearly the job of a physician, but recognition of any unusual or unexpected fluorescence by a knowledgeable photographer during an actual study can

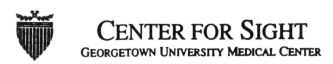

CENTER FOR SIGHT
GEORGETOWN UNIVERSITY MEDICAL CENTER

Informed Consent for Fluorescein Angiography

1. I,   , hereby authorize the
    ophthalmologist or the resident in the Department of
    Ophthalmology at Georgetown University Medical Center
    to administer intravenous fluorescein for the purpose of this
    study as requested by Dr.   .

2. This is a diagnostic study and I understand that no warrant
    or guarantee has been made as to the results or cure.

3. I authorize and direct the aforementioned physician or the
    Georgetown University Medical Center staff to provide such
    additional services as they deem reasonable and necessary.

4. Having received an explanation and given informed consent, I
    hereby agree to release the Georgetown University Medical
    Center, its employees, agents, and medical staff from
    responsibility with regard to permission for this procedure.

    I have read this form carefully before signing it and have been
    given an opportunity to question my physician about this
    procedure.

FORM 6-2. Form for documenting informed consent. (Adapted with permission from Justice J, ed. Ophthalmic Photography. Boston, Mass: Little Brown and Co; 1982.)

prove to be beneficial if the findings are recorded for review by the specialist. In order to know what might be considered out of the ordinary, a photographer should become familiar with fluorescein abnormalities.

Basically, an angiogram is abnormal when there is too much (hyper), too little (hypo), or no fluorescence (Figure 6-12). Late (delayed) fluorescence is also abnormal. On each and every angiogram you perform, try to determine if the study is within or outside normal limits, and why.

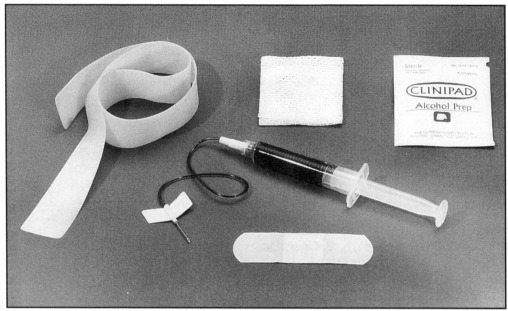

Figure 6-10. Supplies for fluorescein angiography: a tourniquet, fluorescein-filled syringe with a butterfly infusion set, alcohol and gauze pad, and an adhesive bandage.

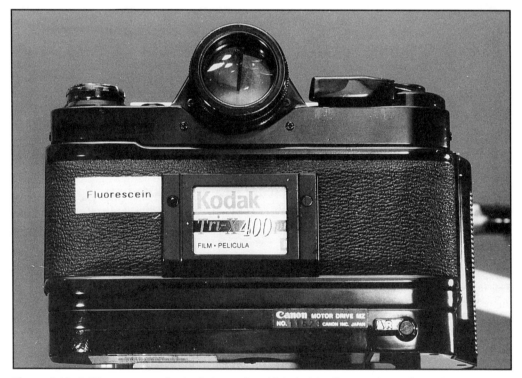

Figure 6-11. A 35-mm camera body designated and labeled for fluorescein angiography.

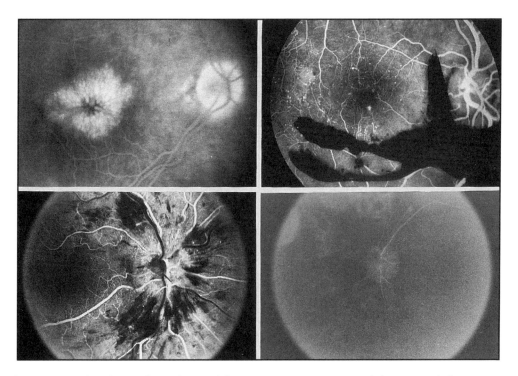

Figure 6-12. Select frames from abnormal fluorescein angiograms. Top left: Too much fluorescence is seen in the macula of this patient with cystoid macular edema. Top right: Too little fluorescence is seen in the portion of the retina being blocked by an overlying vitreous hemorrhage. The patient has proliferative diabetic retinopathy. Bottom left: Delayed venous filling in a patient with a central retinal vein occlusion. Bottom right: A trickle of fluorescein dye is seen in the retinal circulation of this patient with an ophthalmic artery occulsion.

Whenever possible, check your impressions with the interpreting physician. After a while, you will begin to recognize the patterns associated with a particular disease or disorder. As a result, you may find your work more interesting, and you will prove to be a more valuable asset to your employer.

Conclusion

When indicated, fluorescein angiography is a useful diagnostic test for studying the ocular fundi. Experienced fundus photographers, armed with some knowledge of the principles of fluorescence and characteristic flow of dye inside the eye, are usually able to make the transition to fluorescein angiography without difficulty.

References

1. Saine PJ, Bovino JA, Marcus DF, Nelsen PT. Timing of color fundus photographs and intravenous fluorescein angiography. *Am J Ophthalmol.* 1984;97:785.

2. Emerson GA, Anderson HH. Toxicity of certain proposed antileprosy dyes: fluorescein, eosin, erythrosin and others. *Int J Leprosy.* 1934;2:257.

Chapter 7

Slit Lamp Photography

- Slit lamp photos are useful for documenting structural abnormalities and pathological processes.

- Slit lamp illumination can be classified as diffuse, direct, or indirect.

- Illumination techniques may be used alone or in combination.

- For purposes of orientation, first take an overall view of the subject using diffuse illumination and low magnification.

- It is customary to position the light source on the temporal side of the eye being photographed.

Purpose

A slit lamp specifically designed for taking pictures is without rival when it comes to documenting the anterior segment of the eye. Although a suitably equipped hand-held 35-mm camera could be used, a photo slit lamp is preferred since it operates at a more comfortable working distance, provides the user with a moveable source of illumination of changeable size and shape, and offers a wider range of magnification.

Subjects that lend themselves to slit lamp photography are the very same structures that are best examined under the light of a clinical slit lamp—the eyelids, lashes, sclera, conjunctiva, cornea, tear film, anterior chamber, iris, lens, and anterior vitreous. When supplementary lenses are used in combination with special techniques, structures normally hidden from sight (such as the angle of the anterior chamber) can be seen and photographed with a photo slit lamp.

Indications

Because slit lamp photographs are visual records, they are often incorporated into the patient's chart to document structural abnormalities or pathological processes. Participants in clinical research may also be photographed with a slit lamp to help investigators assess the long-term results of an experimental procedure or treatment involving the anterior segment of the eye. Normal ocular anatomy may be photographed for use as illustrations in lectures, journals, or textbooks geared toward the training and education of eyecare professionals.

Patient Education and Orientation

Of the patients referred for slit lamp photography, most will have already been seen by an eye doctor and examined with a slit lamp. Being photographed with one, however, is a little bit different. Lids and lashes, easily ignored when seen through the microscope's eyepiece, are faithfully recorded by the camera. A blink of the eye when the picture is taken results in a blank on film. To get the best results, elicit your patient's cooperation by explaining what you are doing and what you need him or her to do.

What the Patient Needs to Know

- You are not being x-rayed.
- This is simply a microscope with a camera attached.
- Keeping your head and chin in the face rest will help keep your eye in focus.
- You may blink unless asked not to.

Physician's Orders

As with other types of clinical photography, the use of a requisition form is recommended to enhance the communication process between the eye doctor and ocular photographer (FORM 7-1). Providing a place for sketching out the appearance and location of the area to be photographed is helpful, especially when a clear structure like the cornea or crystalline lens is the subject. Subtle findings are easily overlooked unless you know approximately where they are.

CENTER FOR SIGHT
GEORGETOWN UNIVERSITY MEDICAL CENTER

Anterior Segment Photography

Date: _____

Name: _____ DOB: _____ Age: _____ Sex: _____

Physician: _____ Referring Physician: _____

Address: _____

Ocular
Diagnosis: _____ ICD.9 Code(s) _____

Reason for Photos: _____

External Eye Photography:

☐ **Eye Plastic Series**
Head Shot (1:10)
Both Eyes (1:4)
• Primary Position
• Upgaze
• Downgaze
Each Eye (1:2)
• Primary Position

☐ **Orbital Series**
Eye Plastic Series
Worm's Eye View (1:4)

☐ **Nine Positions of Gaze**

☐ **Motility Series**
Head Shot (1:10)
Both Eyes (1:4)
• Primary Position
• Upgaze
• Downgaze
• Looking Left
• Looking Right

☐ **Ptosis Series**
Both Eyes (1:4)
• Primary Position
• Upgaze
• Downgaze

☐ **Other** _____

Slit Lamp Photography:

OD   OS

Eye(s)	Illumination
☐ OD	☐ Diffuse
☐ OS	☐ Direct
☐ OU	☐ Indirect

Specular Microscopy:

Eye(s)	# of Cells
☐ OD	OD OS
☐ OS	
☐ OU	

FORM 7-1. Anterior segment photography form.

Equipment

A photographic slit lamp is basically the same as the instrument used clinically, with a few extras. A camera body, electronic flash, background illuminator, and lens diffuser are attached to the microscope and light source, giving it photographic capability and versatility (Figure 7-1). For a thorough discussion on the slit lamp's use, please refer to the Basic Bookshelf title The Slit Lamp Primer.

The viewing assembly, common to all slit lamps (photographic or otherwise), is much like an ordinary microscope, except that it is turned on its side to face the patient. Its purpose is to magnify that which is not easily seen with the naked eye. For lighting, an illumination source designed specifically for looking at eyes is coupled with the microscope. Although this light is a medical device, it operates much like the spots used to light a Broadway stage or Hollywood set.

A theatrical spotlight produces a circular beam of illumination when its metal flaps, called barn doors, are opened. By changing the position of these flaps, the shape of the projected light is altered and the beam size reduced (Figure 7-2). The light of the slit lamp can also be modified with its own internal barn door-like components. By turning the appropriate knobs or controls, its beam can be shaped into a circle, slit, or moon of various sizes (Figure 7-3).

To change the amount and quality of light from a spotlight, a piece of fabric called a scrim is placed in front of its lamp (Figure 7-4). This light diffuser will reduce the lamp's effective intensity and soften the edges of the shadows. When a diffuser is placed over the light of the slit lamp, it will also be less intense, and the shadows will soften as a result of the light spreading out.

The slit lamp microscope and illuminator are designed to work together as a unit, even though both are able to move independently. Because they swing on the same axis (copivotal), they will focus on the same plane (parfocal) and, at the same time, keep the slit beam centered in the field (isocentric) so long as this relationship is maintained.

Lighting

Although a myriad of illumination methods are available with a photo slit lamp, light emanating from this instrument can be classified primarily as either diffuse, direct, or indirect. Each of these three types of illumination may be used alone or in combination. The nature of the photographic subject will dictate the specific type of lighting to use.

Diffuse Illumination

When the cloud layer is dense enough to completely obscure the sun, we experience a natural form of diffuse illumination. On such a day our world lacks contrast, and most shadows are absent because of the overcast sky. A beam of light from the slit lamp will soften when a diffusion lens is placed over it, producing an artificial form of diffuse illumination. This low-contrast light is shadowless and well-suited for the overall inspection of the eye and its surroundings (Figure 7-5).

Direct Illumination

Sunlight on a cloudless day provides the brightest, most contrasty form of natural light. Shadows are dense and sharply defined when the sun is overhead and the sky is clear. Without a diffusion lens, the light beam from the slit lamp is also sharp and focused and is used to directly illuminate the subject (Figure 7-6). By adjusting an internal aperture, the size and shape of the beam can be changed from a full circle to a pinpoint of light or from a narrow sliver to a broad beam of illumination (Figure 7-7). Regardless of its size or shape, a light pointed right at an object will light it directly.

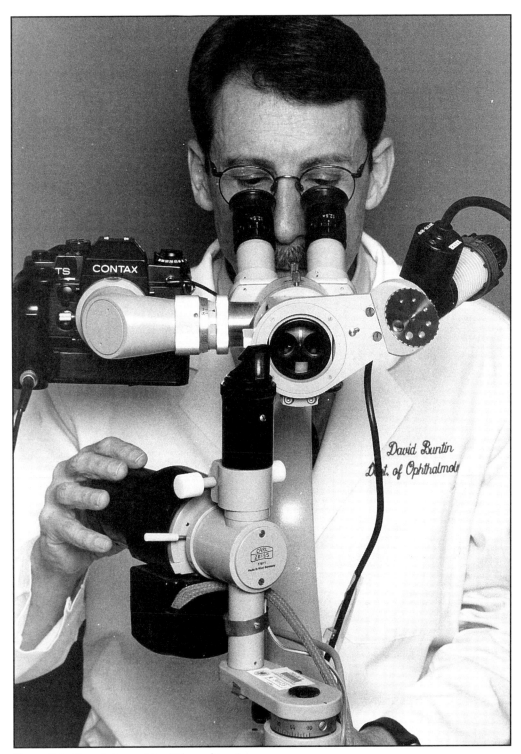

Figure 7-1. The photographic slit lamp biomicroscope.

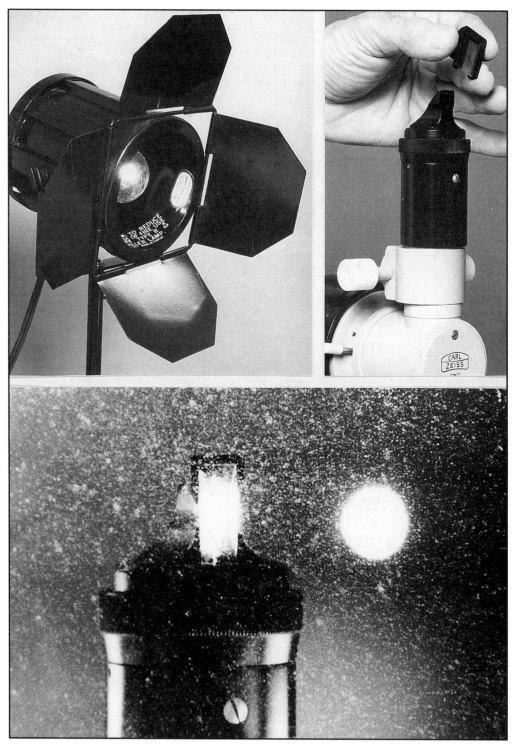

Figure 7-2. Top left: A Hollywood-type spotlight with its barn doors open and diffusion screen off. Top right: The light from a slit lamp can be used as a spotlight once its diffuser is removed. Bottom: A focused spot of light from the slit lamp is well seen on this piece of lightly dusted glass.

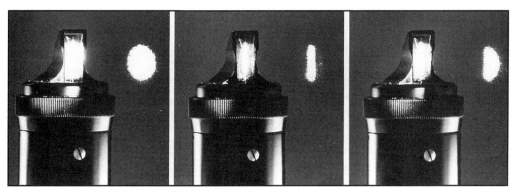

Figure 7-3. The different shapes of the beam of light from a slit lamp illuminator.

Narrow Beam

When the slit beam is shaped into a sliver, it can be used to illuminate an optical section of the eye. This narrow knife of light is often used to localize changes in various layers of the cornea.

Broad Beam

A wide, broad beam of light is more effective than a narrow slit in demonstrating the extent to which an area has been affected.

Tangential

Placing light off to the side of an eye (but still aimed and centered on it) is a good technique for accentuating surface texture. This type of lighting, called tangential illumination, is most effective in emphasizing the nooks and crannies of a structure (Figure 7-8), so it is often used to view and photograph the iris.

Pinpoint

Cells and flare (signs of infection) in the aqueous can be seen easily with a small circle of light, but they are very difficult to capture photographically because of their low reflectivity. Consequently, pinpoint illumination is used most often by the clinician, not the photographer.

Specular Reflection

An object that reflects light bends it back to the observer. When the reflecting surface is polished or smooth, like a body of still water, the reflection looks almost real, and it may be difficult to tell the reflected object from the actual item (Figure 7-9). Reflections with mirror-like qualities are called specular reflections.

The specular reflection of the slit lamp's main light source is well seen on the smooth surface of the cornea (Figure 7-10). During routine photography, it is best to de-emphasize this highlight so it does not get in the way and mask any underlying pathology.

For visualization of the corneal endothelial cell layer, however, this reflection must not only be found, but also enhanced (Figure 7-11) as these cells are best seen just adjacent to the brightest part of the reflection when using a narrow slit beam.

To accentuate this all important specular reflection, position the slit lamp's microscope and illumination source about 60° apart.[1-3] This is easily achieved by separately placing both the microscope and the illuminator approximately 30° off the axis of fixation. Once these two components are placed at opposite and equal angles to the corneal surface and the reflection is seen,

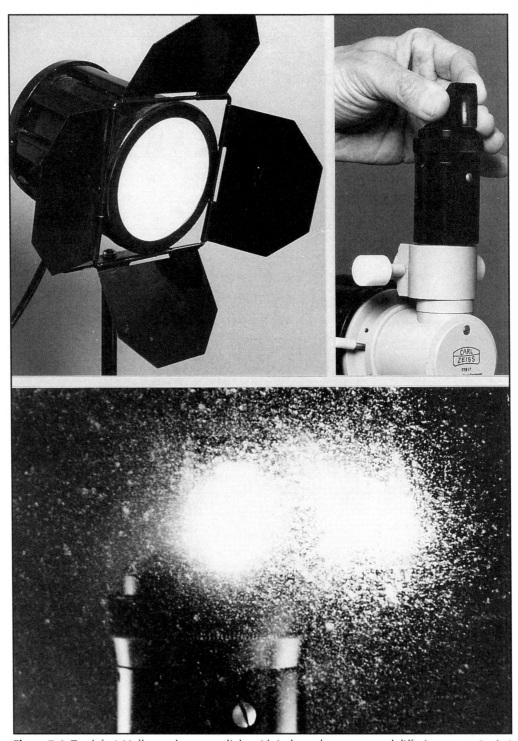

Figure 7-4. Top left: A Hollywood-type spotlight with its barn doors open and diffusion screen (scrim) in place. Top right: The light from the slit lamp will soften and spread when a diffuser is placed over its illumination source. Bottom: A diffuse beam of light from the slit lamp is well seen on this lightly dusted piece of glass. (Compare to Figure 7-2.)

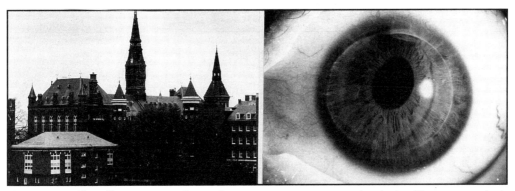

Figure 7-5. Diffuse illumination. Left: A college campus at noon on a cloudy day. There are no shadows. Right: A left eye photographed by the diffused light of a slit lamp. This soft type of lighting is good for a general inspection of the eye.

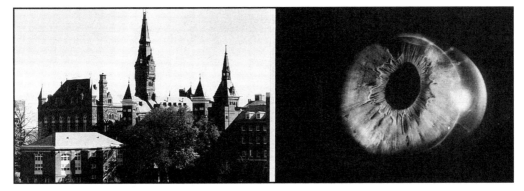

Figure 7-6. Direct illumination (compare to Figure 7-5). Left: A college campus at noon on a cloudless, sunny day. Notice the many shadows present. Right: A left eye photographed with the circular beam of the slit lamp. The diffusion lens was not used. Notice how the subject is isolated with this "spotlight."

the cells are focused by careful and deliberate manipulation of the joy stick and/or the patient's eye. Because the endothelial cells are tiny, the microscope's magnification must be set to the maximum (Figure 7-12) if they are to be visible in the final photographic print or slide.

Examining the corneal endothelial cell layer with a slit lamp is not easy. Taking sharp pictures of this single cell layer is even more difficult because the normal microsaccadic movement of the eyes, exaggerated by the high magnification, cause the pictures to blur. Because of this, an ordinary photo slit lamp is not often used to photograph this cellular layer. When photographs are desired, a specular microscope with photographic capability (Figure 7-13) is generally used.

Indirect Illumination

If you direct a sharply focused beam of light at the central cornea of a patient wearing a contact lens, the contact will seem to disappear. Aim the light beam off to the side of the eye, at the limbus instead, and the contact lens will reappear, almost magically. Transparent objects and ocular structures are often better visualized by such indirect methods of illumination.

In its normal position, the slit lamp illuminator is centered directly on the object under examination, and its beam will appear in the middle of every photograph. For most types of indirect illumination (Figure 7-14), however, the light needs to be directed away from the subject. To

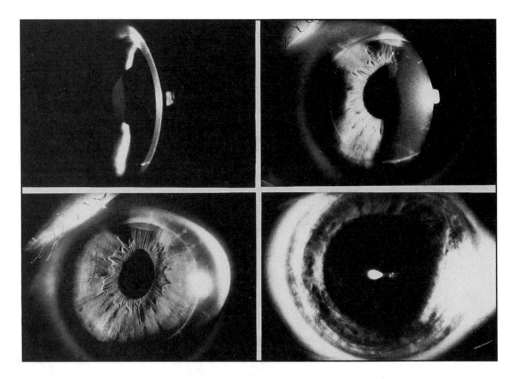

Figure 7-7. Examples of direct illumination with the slit lamp. (All photos except bottom right are of the left eye of a patient who had a corneal transplant for Keratoconus.) Top left: A narrow beam. Top right: A broad beam. Bottom left: A full circle of light placed tangentially. Bottom right: A small circle, or pinpoint, of light was used to demonstrate the changes in the transparency of the aqueous.

achieve this, the isocentric relationship between the microscope and the illuminator must be broken. This is done by moving the appropriate knob in the desired direction (Figure 7-15) until the light is decentered sufficiently.

Proximal

A light placed near a problem area, rather than directly over it, can sometimes be the most effective way to highlight it. This proximal type of illumination should be considered when directly lighting the area is not providing the view you need.

Sclerotic Scatter

Changes in the cornea are difficult to light directly because of the transparent nature of the structure. When light is instead aimed at the sclera (near the limbus) of that same eye, even subtle changes can often be well delineated.

Retroillumination

When a source of light illuminates a subject from behind, it is seen in silhouette. This type of lighting is most effective when light reflected from the retina or iris is used to outline the shape of a lesion in the patient's lens or cornea.

Transillumination

A structure that is normally opaque can exhibit transillumination defects when a light is shone

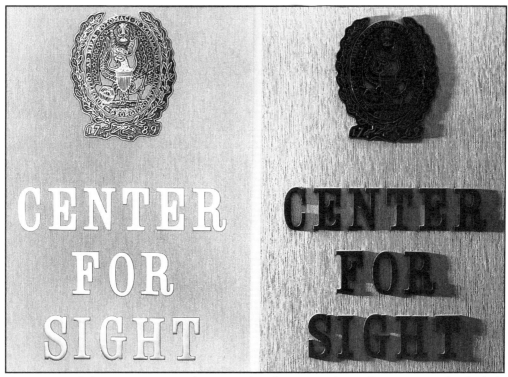

Figure 7-8. A lighting comparison of a textured surface using direct illumination. Left: The light source was placed in front of the subject. Right: The light source was tangentially placed to the left side of the subject. Notice that as the light skims the surface, the texture of the wall and the raised letters become more obvious.

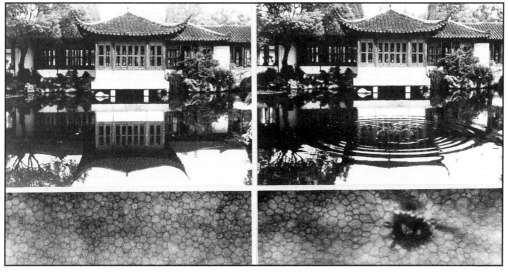

Figure 7-9. Specular reflections. Top left: Both the subject and its reflection are well seen in this Chinese museum. Top right: When the stillness of the water is disturbed, the reflection is also affected. Bottom left: A reflection of an intact corneal endothelium. Bottom right: A reflection of a disturbed area of the endothelium in an eye with Fuch's corneal dystrophy.

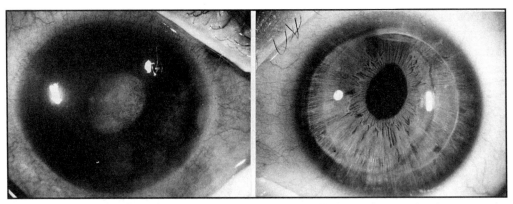

Figure 7-10. Two distinct corneal reflections may be seen in a slit lamp photograph. The rectangular reflection is from the main illumination source, while the circular highlight is from the background illuminator. Left: The disruption of the specular reflections in this glaucomatous right eye may be a cause for concern. Right: The sharp and clear specular reflections seen in this left eye following a penetrating keratoplasty suggest that the cornea is healthy.

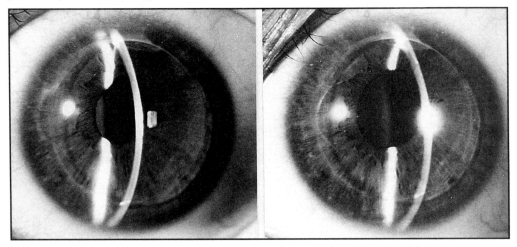

Figure 7-11. A narrow slit beam. Left: With the central rectangular reflection of the light source de-emphasized. Right: With the central rectangular reflection of the light source enhanced.

through it. Whether a disease process or surgical procedure is responsible for the problem, transillumination can highlight the involved areas.

Background Illumination

A slit lamp designed for photographic purposes is usually equipped with a background light. Such a light is most helpful when used in conjunction with a narrow slit beam, which provides orientation for the viewer (Figure 7-16).

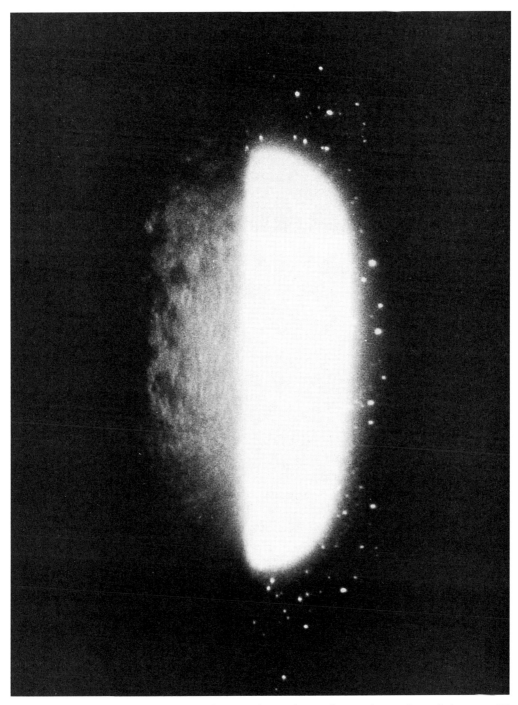

Figure 7-12. The corneal endothelium of a normal eye taken with an ordinary photo slit lamp at 40X magnification.

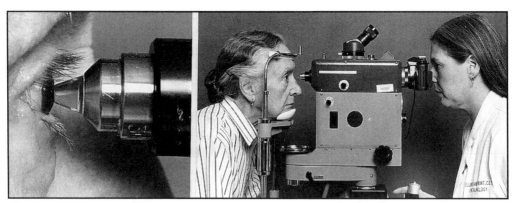

Figure 7-13. A contact specular microscope.

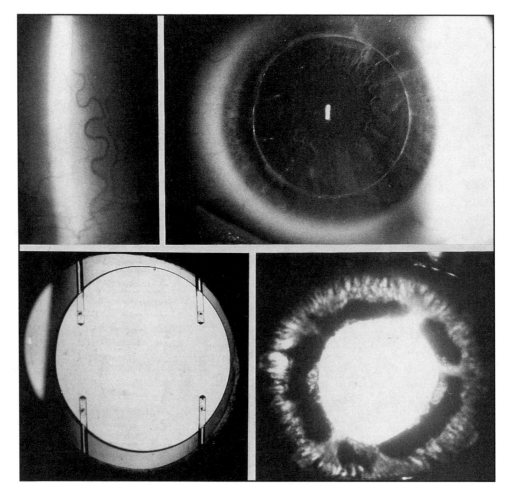

Figure 7-14. Examples of indirect illumination. Top left: Proximal illumination of a scleral blood vessel. Top right: Sclerotic scatter was used to highlight the circular surgical scar after a successful corneal transplant. Bottom left: Retroillumination from the fundus was used effectively to highlight this posterior chamber intraocular lens. Bottom right: Transillumination demonstrates iris atrophy.

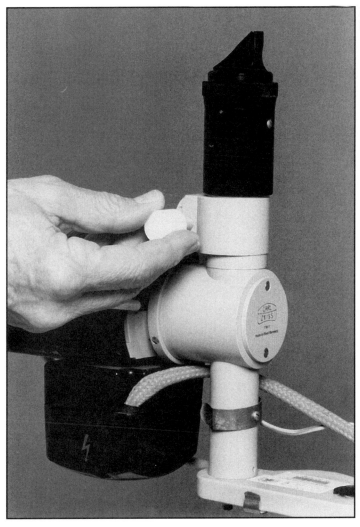

Figure 7-15. Decentering the beam of light.

Technique

For purposes of orientation, it is helpful to first take an overall view of the subject using diffuse illumination at a low magnification. This is important for differentiating between the right and left eye, particularly when the subject is very small or lacks normal landmarks. Next, isolate the area of interest by selecting an appropriate magnification and lighting technique. Diffuse illumination is good for a generalized ocular inspection, but direct and indirect illumination are better at highlighting a specific problem.

When a slit beam is used, it is customary to place the illumination source on the temporal side of the eye being photographed so the base of the curved slit faces the patient's nose. That way the light placement is not limited by the nose. Standardizing the position of the light source is also helpful in identifying the right eye from the left in a slit lamp photograph (Figure 7-17).

In general, more than one picture will be needed to accurately represent the subject, and more than one form of illumination will be used. Although visual experimentation is one way to decide how you will light an eye, having a mental menu of the most common forms of illumination will help insure that you don't forget any obvious choices.

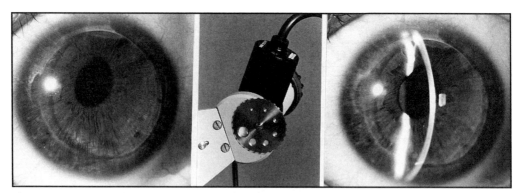

Figure 7-16. Center: The background illumination source. Left: Used alone. Right: Used in combination with a narrow slit beam.

A Mnemonic for Slit Lamp Illumination

As a grammar school student (and horrible speller), I was delighted to learn a recall phrase that made spelling a difficult word easy. To spell arithmetic, I simply memorized the mnemonic "a rat in the house might eat the ice cream." The first letter of each word spelled arithmetic.

Mnemonics aren't just for kids. After many years of haphazardly applying whatever lighting technique I happened upon, I found that memorizing a recall phrase of a short list of illumination types was the only way for me to gain consistency and positive results with my slit lamp photography (Table 7-1).

Film Selection

As with other types of medical photography, the slit lamp camera is usually loaded with color transparency film. Depending on the output of the flash, a slow, medium, or high speed may be chosen. To keep it simple, you may wish to use the same film that you use to take fundus photographs.

If your slit lamp has adjustable f-stops, select a film that allows you to use smaller apertures in order to take advantage of an increased depth of field. Don't forget to consider your patient when choosing a particular film. If the camera's flash is powerful enough for a very slow film to be used (ISO 25), but the light from the flash blows your patient out of his or her seat, perhaps obtaining the highest quality photograph is in direct conflict with your job as a health care provider. After all, the comfort of the patient must be paramount.

If prints are needed for publication, a B&W film may be used instead of color since illustrations in scientific journals and texts are printed in black and white. When both color and B&W pictures are needed, shoot the subject only on color film to save the patient from unnecessary discomfort. An experienced darkroom technician can make internegatives from the slides in order to obtain the necessary B&W prints.

Conclusion

All the conventional slit lamp examination and illumination techniques can be achieved with

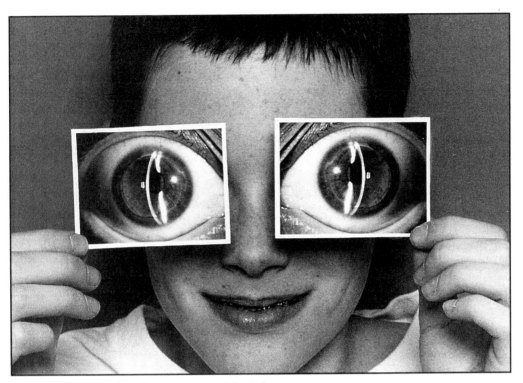

Figure 7-17. Standardize the positioning of the light source.

the photo slit lamp. Because slit lamp photography is difficult, proficiency with the instrument—with or without a camera attached—is a must. Fortunately, all the conventional examination and illumination techniques used clinically may be applied photographically.

References

1. Coppinger JM, Maio M, Miller K. *Ophthalmic Photography*. Thorofare, NJ: SLACK Incorporated; 1988:54.
2. Martoyni CL, Bahn CF, and Meyer RF. Clinical slit lamp biomicroscopy and photo slit lamp biomicrography. *Journal of Ophthalmic Photography*. 1984;7:28.
3. Wong D. *Textbook of Ophthalmic Photography*. Birmingham, Ala: Inter-optics Publications, Inc; 1982:46.

Table 7-1

A MNEMONIC FOR SLIT LAMP ILLUMINATION

DIFFUSE	Doctors,
DIRECT	Do
Narrow	not
Broad Beam	boldly
Tangential	touch
Pinpoint	patients'
Specular Reflection	spines.
INDIRECT	Ideally,
Proximal	patients
Sclerotic Scatter	should
Retroillumination	rest
Transillumination	today.

Chapter 8

Photographic Organization

- Data on every patient who is photographed should be recorded in a photography log.

- Patient ID can be recorded on film by photographing an area of the requisition form, using an internal ID tag, or using a film check tab.

- Photos and slides should be labeled with essential information.

- The position and appearance of the macula, optic nerve, and blood vessels can be used to orient the viewer of retinal photographs.

- No matter how perfect a photograph is, if it can't be located, it is worthless.

Overseeing a collection of clinical photographs entails more than just filing the pictures away in a desk drawer. Images must be readily available for inspection (or interpretation), which requires that an efficient system be in place to identify, store, and retrieve a patient's pictures. Ideally, such a system blends the demands of the users with available resources so that the photographs are convenient to access and affordable to maintain.

RA

The Photography Log

A record should be kept listing every patient who is photographed. It doesn't matter whether the details of the patient's visit are handwritten in a log book or entered into a computer database. Either method works well. The important thing is that essential information is obtained and permanently recorded.

What is regarded as essential information will vary from one clinic to another. Unless your photographs are filed by medical record number, however, the patient's name is usually the most important piece of data collected for photographic record keeping. The patient's record number, date of birth, sex, and doctor are often noted, along with the date of the patient's visit. Sometimes a medical diagnosis is recorded as well as the type of pictures taken and the specific eye photographed. Whatever information is deemed important in your practice is essential, and should be gathered and entered in the photographic log. If your records are handwritten, legibility is crucial.

The Requisition Form

Essential information can be obtained from the patient's chart, but it is more efficient to have all necessary details written out on a photographic requisition form (FORM 8-1). Such a form provides the ordering physician with a way to spell out exactly what he or she requires of the photographer. If designed well, this requisition can also double as a patient identification (ID) tag when the appropriate information is grouped together on the form and photographed.

For use as an ID tag, the area of the form containing essential information must be photographed on the same roll of film and on the frame immediately preceding the clinical photographs. This ID photo is especially valuable when the person labeling the pictures is not the photographer.

To obtain an ID photo of the requisition with the equipment used in external eye photography, just aim, focus, and shoot. Do the same when using the fundus camera (Figure 8-1) or photo slit lamp. Some fundus cameras provide a tiny plastic slate for use as a name tag. This is inserted into the camera and photographed along with the eye itself. As long as the tag is in the camera, the name written on it will appear in each and every picture taken (Figure 8-2). If you are using a requisition form, there is no need to use this type of ID card. In addition, having a readable name on a clinical photograph is problematic if the images are to be shown in public. A person's right to privacy must always be respected, so identifiable images must not be displayed without the patient's permission.

Using the requisition form as an ID tag can be a problem if your camera system magnifies the subject too much. Some slit lamp cameras, even when set to their lowest power, can enlarge the patient's name and date so much that letters are chopped off, making the information unreadable (Figure 8-3). If the doctor filling out the form is able to write very small, it's possible that this system can be salvaged, but it is unlikely. Asking that a form be filled out legibly is one thing,

PENNSTATE

College of Medicine
University Hospital · Children's Hospital
The Milton S. Hershey Medical Center

OPHTHALMIC PHOTOGRAPHY REQUEST FORM

Date: _____

Name: _____   Age: ____ Sex: ____ Patient Number: _____

Ordering Physician: _____   Referring Physician: _____

Address: _____

OCULAR DIAGNOSIS: _____

Reason for Photos: _____

VISUAL ACUITY	MEDIA OPACITY		SYSTEMIC DISEASE

VISUAL ACUITY

RE _____

LE _____

I.O.P.

RE _____

LE _____

MEDIA OPACITY

Cornea   ☐ RE ☐ LE
Lens   ☐ RE ☐ LE
Vitreous   ☐ RE ☐ LE

APHAKIC   ☐ RE ☐ LE
PSEUDOPHAKIC ☐ RE ☐ LE

SYSTEMIC DISEASE

☐ Diabetes
☐ Hypertension
☐ Other _____

DRUG THERAPY

☐ Insulin
☐ INH
☐ Chloroquine
☐ Epinephrine
☐ Ethambutol
☐ Anticoagulant

VISUAL FIELD (comment) _____

EYE SURGERY _____

ALLERGY _____

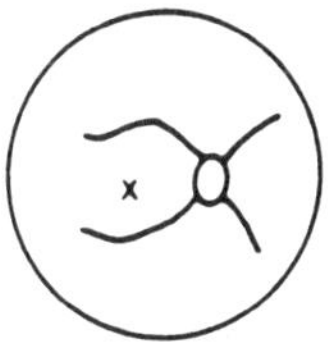

STANDARD PHOTOGRAPHIC FIELDS

Field 1 - Disc
Field 2 - Macula
Field 3 - Temporal to macula
Field 4 - Superior temporal
Field 5 - Inferior temporal
Field 6 - Superior nasal
Field 7 - Inferior nasal

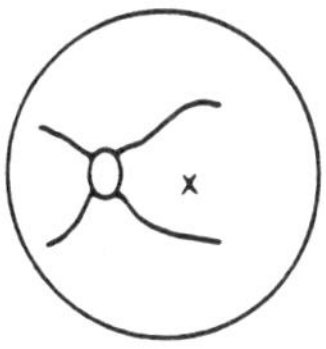

RIGHT EYE   LEFT EYE

FLUORESCEIN ANGIOGRAPHY ONLY

Transit:

Which eye: right   left

What field: _____

Late views:

Which eye(s): right   left   both

What field(s): _____

PHOTOGRAPHIC PROCEDURES OTHER THAN I.V.F.A.

☐ Color fundus photography

☐ Stereo disc photos

☐ External photography

☐ Slit lamp photos

☐ Nerve fiber layer (B&W)

Which eye(s):

right   left   both

What field(s):
☐ Disc
☐ Macula
☐ 7 fields
☐ Other

FORM 8-1. An ophthalmic photography requisition form.

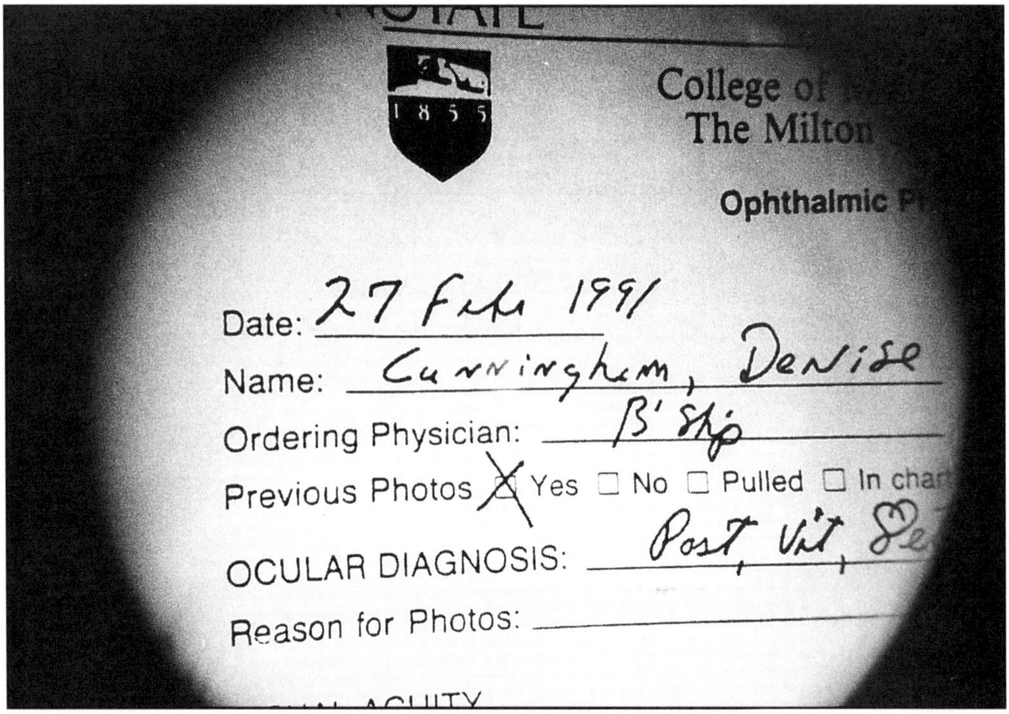

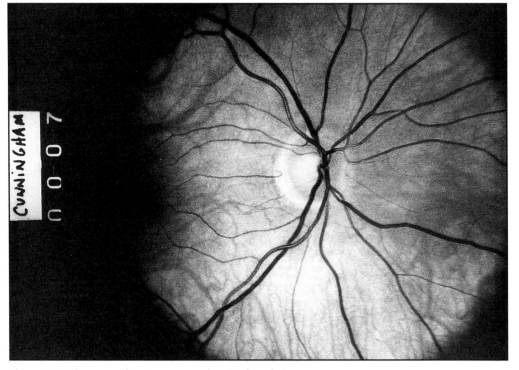

Figure 8-1. The top portion of a photographic requisition form well designed to serve as an ID tag. This was photographed with a fundus camera.

Figure 8-2. The name slate tag was used to ID this photo.

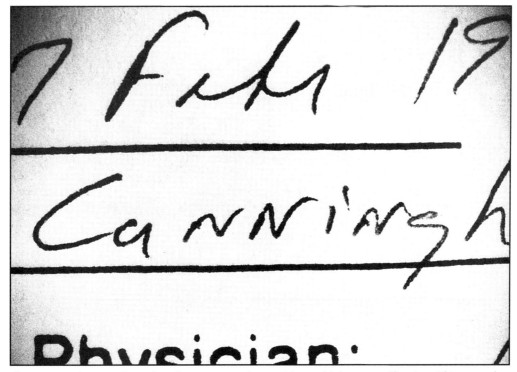

Figure 8-3. Photographing the photo request form with too high a magnification. This was photographed with a slit lamp camera.

insisting that it be written as small as possible is quite another matter. In this case, a film check tab may be the answer.

Film check tabs are self-stick labels that allow individual rolls of film to be easily identified for special handling or processing. You've seen these tabs before on film developed commercially. Usually check tabs are found on the photo envelope or glued to a negative strip, but they may appear in other places. If you've ever tried to squeeze an extra picture out of a 36-exposure roll of film, you may be disappointed to find a film check tab stuck right on your 37th exposure (Figure 8-4).

While commercial photofinishers utilize film check tabs in large numbers, small quantities of these labels can be purchased for use by the occasional user (Figure 8-5). Manufacturers generally require a minimum order of thousands of labels, but photographic equipment catalogs will often sell rolls of 100 twin-numbered check tabs.

When a film check tab is placed on a photo request form and photographed, it is large enough to read yet small enough to photograph in its entirety (Figure 8-6), making identification easy. After the film has been sorted by film check number, the patient's name can be found by matching the number in the ID photo with the number on the requisition form.

On cameras that feature a small slate for the patient's name, a film check tab can easily be used. Just stick the tab directly onto the ID slate and insert it into the appropriate camera port. The tab will be photographed along with the patient's eye (Figure 8-7).

A specular microscope designed to be used in direct contact with the patient's eye comes equipped with an applanation lens, which does not allow for the conventional recording of written information. As a result, photographing the request form or film check tab is impossible with this instrument. In this case, using two identically numbered film checks may be helpful. One half

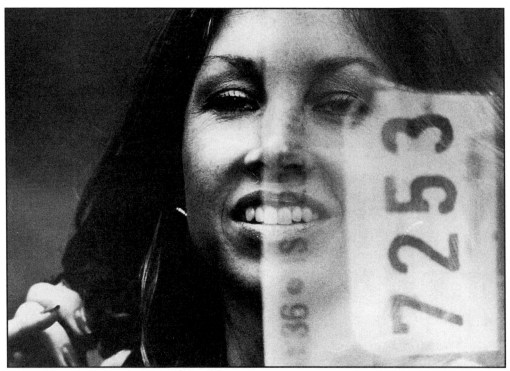

Figure 8-4. The image of a film check tab superimposed on a 35-mm color slide.

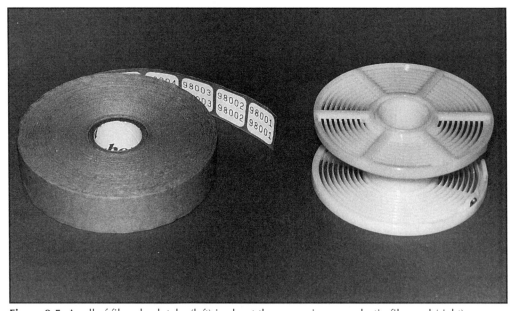

Figure 8-5. A roll of film check tabs (left) is about the same size as a plastic film reel (right).

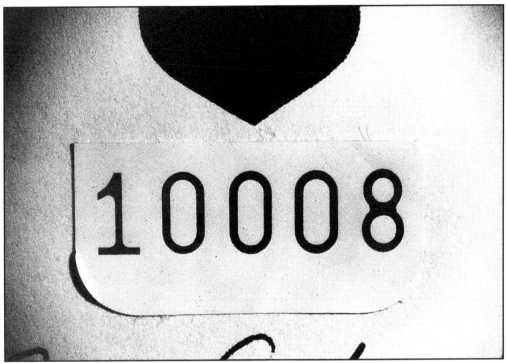

Figure 8-6. An individual film check tab attached to an ophthalmic photography request form. This was photographed with a photo slit lamp.

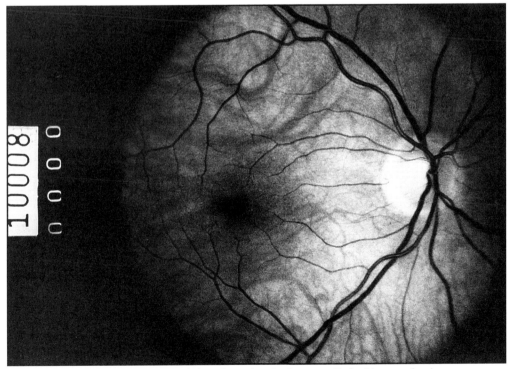

Figure 8-7. A film check tab applied directly to the ID slate supplied with some fundus cameras.

of the pair is affixed to the requisition form while its mate is placed directly on the film itself. These tabs are designed to withstand the wet conditions present during film processing. Once dry, the roll of film can be identified by matching the numbered check with its other half.

Some specular microscopes have specialized camera backs that are capable of imprinting data directly onto the negative. With these cameras, it helps to imprint the film check number (or a portion of it) on the film for purposes of identification and labeling (Figure 8-8).

Labeling

Medical records must be identifiable, and ophthalmic photographs are no exception. All the essential information collected on each patient and entered in the log need not appear on the individual images, but the patient's name and date should be marked somewhere on the print or slide. Fortunately, the cardboard or plastic mounts that frame 35 mm color transparencies provide enough space for recording such important information (Figure 8-9).

External Eye Photographs

In addition to name and date, the viewer is more easily oriented if a directional grid is included on photographs demonstrating positions of gaze. Such a grid is used to show where the patient was attempting to look when the picture was taken. Having this grid stamped on all pictures in a series is also helpful for quick retrieval of a specific image in the absence of a lighted view box (Figure 8-10). Without looking at each and every picture, the appropriate view can be selected based on the grid stamped on its slide mount.

Fundus Photographs

To avoid inadvertently transposing fundus photographs, all should be labeled right or left (R or L, or OD or OS). It is fairly easy to tell the eyes apart when looking at a picture of the front of the eye, but without proper training, a person viewing the inside of an eye may have difficulty distinguishing a right eye from a left eye (Figure 8-11). Learning the normal appearance and placement of basic ocular fundi structures will make proper identification easier and is essential for those who are responsible for labeling these visual medical records.

The landmarks of the inner eye are the macula, optic disc, and retinal blood vessels (Figure 8-12). The macula is the central area of the retina, approximately 1.5 mm in size, oval in shape, and usually darker than its surroundings. This is the part of the eye where vision is sharpest; it is also the area being tested when we measure visual acuity.

The optic disc, the anterior portion of the optic nerve, is the most prominent intraocular structure. It also measures about 1.5 mm in diameter and is located nasally and slightly superior to a horizontal line drawn through the center of the macula. Retinal vessels emerge from and return through the center of this nearly round landmark.

The retinal blood vessels serve well as a tool for orientation inside the fundus. After the central retinal artery enters the inner eye through the optic nerve, it divides above and below the disc on both the nasal and temporal sides to form four separate branches. These branches transport blood that nourishes the four quadrants of the retina. The blood then makes its way through smaller arterioles and capillaries, then through venules and veins until it leaves the eye through the central retinal vein at the optic nerve.

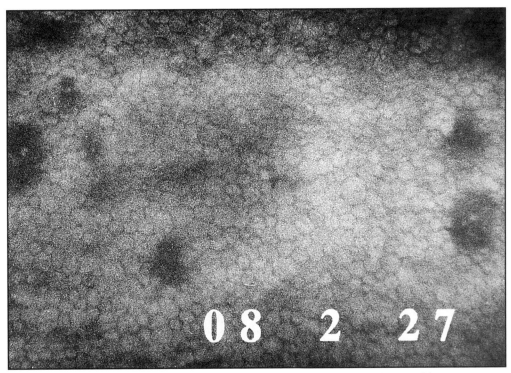

Figure 8-8. When a specialized 35 mm camera data back is used, it may be possible to print numbers directly onto the film. In this case, consider using the number of the film check tab along with the date the picture was taken. The numbers "08" in this photograph of the corneal endothelium are the last two digits of film check #10008. The "2 27" represents the month and day that the photograph was taken.

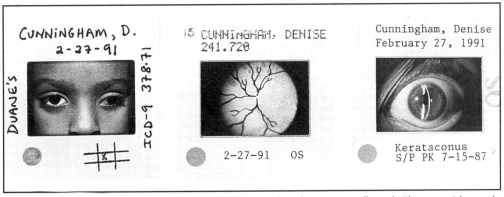

Figure 8-9. Mounts for 35-mm transparency film may be plastic or cardboard. They provide ample space for recording essential information that may be handwritten (left), imprinted directly on the slide (middle), or typed onto labels, which are then affixed to the slide (right). Always be sure to double check your spelling before affixing labels to your slides.

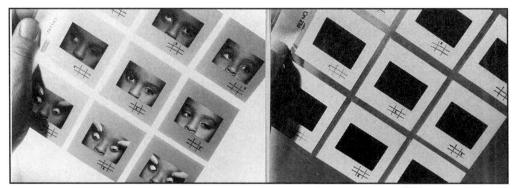

Figure 8-10. Marking a directional grid on the slide mount makes it easy to sort through slides showing positions of gaze even if a lighted view box is unavailable.

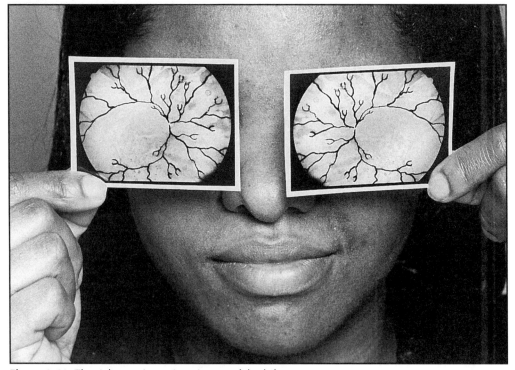

Figure 8-11. The right eye is a mirror image of the left eye.

Because the temporal retinal vessels curve, or arch, around the macula, they are often referred to as the superior temporal and inferior temporal arcades. In comparison, the nasal branches of the retinal arteries and veins are straight. Remembering this can provide a valuable clue for orientation when a retinal photograph contains neither the macula nor the disc. If the major blood vessels in the picture are curved, you're probably viewing the temporal retina, above or below the macula. If these vessels are straight, chances are, you are nasal to the optic nerve.

The angle formed where the blood vessels divide can also help you orient yourself inside the eye. The acute angles created by the bifurcations of smaller blood vessels point, like arrows, toward larger branches which, in turn, point toward the optic disc. Just as all branches on a tree point towards its trunk, all retinal blood vessels point toward the disc (Figure 8-13).

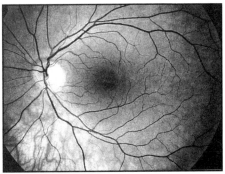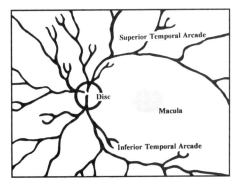

Figure 8-12. The landmarks of the ocular fundus include the disc, macula, and temporal arcades. Left: A monochromatic fundus photograph of a normal left eye. Right: A graphic representation of the landmarks of a left fundus.

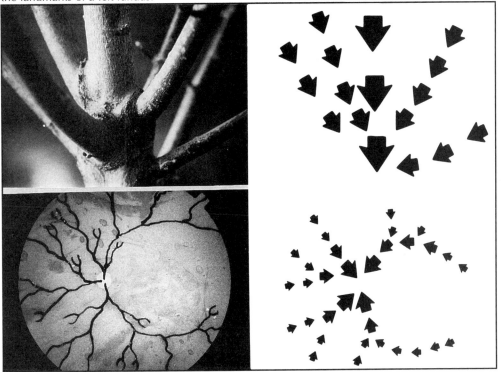

Figure 8-13. The branches of a tree point toward its trunk just as the blood vessels of the retina (model eye) point toward its "trunk", the optic nerve.

Fluorescein Angiograms

RA

The contact sheet of a fluorescein angiogram needs to be labeled with the usual information, such as name and date of the study (Figure 8-14).

Slit Lamp Photographs

It is fairly easy to distinguish a right eye from a left eye on photographs taken under diffuse illumination using low magnification. When direct illumination is employed, or when the subject is highly magnified, it may be impossible to tell one eye from the other. Because of this, it is recommended that at least one picture in the series of every eye photographed with the slit lamp

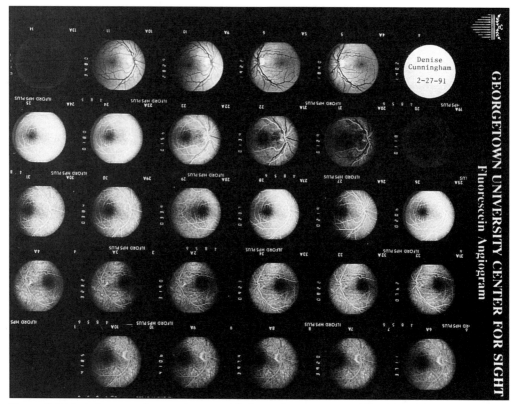

Figure 8-14. Label a print of an angiogram with the patient's name and the date of the study. If space permits, include your company or institutional logo on this photograph.

camera be taken with diffuse lighting at low magnification.

Standardizing the placement of the specular reflection of both the illumination source and background light can also help the viewer know which eye is which. The custom is to place the reflection from the main light on the temporal aspect of the eye and put the background illuminator's reflection nearest the patient's nose. When using a narrow slit beam, it is also useful to light the eye temporally so that the C-shaped beam of light bends toward the patient's nose (Figure 8-15). Of course, if the patient's pathology prevents such placement, light the eye to best demonstrate the subject matter.

Specular Micrographs

The size, shape, and density of corneal endothelial cells often show how well this single layer of cells is functioning. In the adult, normal cell counts range from approximately 1500-2000/mm^2. Because the corneal endothelium does not replicate, an eye with a cell count of less than 500/mm^2 may be at risk for corneal decompensation from edema. Specular microscopy is a good way to assess the integrity of the endothelium.

Corneal endothelial cell density is obtained by counting the number of cells present in representative photographic views of the cornea and averaging the results. Counting cells is often done by placing a transparent grid overlay on a photographic enlargement of the subject. Superimposing the grid directly on the print (Figure 8-16) allows the viewer to verify the count. It may also be a more effective method for insuring that the essential information is accurate and available to all who review the pictures.

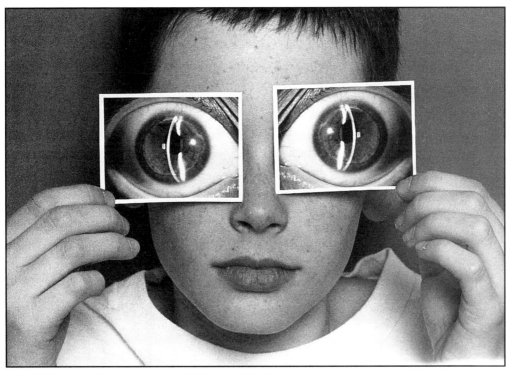

Figure 8-15. Standardize the placement of the slit lamp's reflection on the cornea.

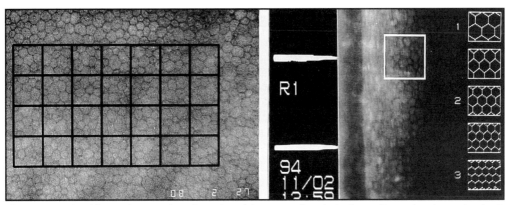

Figure 8-16. A grid superimposed on the print of the corneal endothelium allows the viewer to check the cell density. Left: A photograph taken with a contact microscope. Right: A photograph taken with a non-contact device.

`RA`

Storage

After processing, all photographic film must be safely protected to avoid damaging its fragile emulsion. The ideal storage system should both protect the negatives and transparencies from mishandling and allow the viewers easy access to them. In the past, securing such storage was sometimes difficult, so it was not unusual to see slides grouped by a rubber band or secured to a progress note with ordinary adhesive tape. Fortunately, with the availability of inexpensive and safe storage materials, such improvisation is no longer necessary.

Black and white negatives should be cut into manageable strips and placed in storage envelopes or pages. Clear holders are considered superior since negatives need not be removed for review. Because they are taken out only for printing, handling is kept to a minimum.

Color transparencies must also be appropriately protected. After they are properly labeled, they should be stored in protective plastic sheets, boxes, or drawers designed specifically for this purpose. With individual storage sheets, you have the option of placing the photographic images directly into the patient's chart for maximum accessibility.

Clinical images may be kept in the patient's chart or filed separately. A simple three-ring binder system with negative sleeves and slide pages filed alphabetically or numerically works well in a small practice, but a separate photographic chart may be needed if the photographic collection is expansive.

`RA`

Retrieval

To insure patient confidentiality, access to medical records must be limited to authorized personnel. If filed separately from the chart, a patient's photographs must be protected from unauthorized browsers. A designated file area or room with appropriate safeguards is usually effective.

`OptA`

`OphA`

Properly filed images are easy to locate. You open the appropriate drawer and pull out the desired chart or envelope. Retrieval is difficult when images have not yet been placed in the file cabinet. This is where a well-designed log book or computer program will show its true worth.

In an efficient system, each and every roll of film of the same type will go through the process in the very same order and have its progress documented in the log. Knowing when a roll of film has been developed, labeled, reviewed, or filed makes tracking a missing roll easy. Design your photographic log with these valuable entries in mind.

Conclusion

The quick labeling of clinical photographs with essential information allows for easy and accurate identification. With an efficient filing system and a well-maintained photographic log, rapid retrieval of these medical records is simplified. After all, no matter how well a photographer captures the subject on film, if the pictures cannot be found, they are worthless.

Bibliography

Allen L. Slit-lamp biomicrography. In: Justice J Jr, ed. *Ophthalmic Photography.* Boston, Mass: Little, Brown and Co; 1982.

Behrendt T, Wilson LA. Spectral reflectance photography of the retina. *Am J Ophthalmol.* 1965;59:1080-1088.

Berliner ML. *Biomicroscopy of the Eye.* New York, NY: Paul B. Hoeber, Inc; 1943.

Brooks DB. *Lenses and Lens Accessories.* Somerville, Mass: Curtin and London, Inc; 1982.

Busse BJ, Mittleman D. Use of the astigmatism correction device on the Zeiss fundus camera for peripheral retinal photography. In: Justice J, Jr, ed. *Ophthalmic Photography.* Boston, Mass: Little, Brown, and Co; 1982:65-76.

Coppinger JM, Maio M, Miller K. *Ophthalmic Photography.* Thorofare, NJ: SLACK Incorporated; 1988.

Curtin D, DeMaio J. *The Darkroom Handbook.* New York, NY: Curtin and London, Inc; 1979.

Delori FC, Gragoudas ES. Examination of the ocular fundus with monochromatic illumination. *Annals of Ophthalmology.* 1976;703-709.

Eaton GT. *Photographic Chemistry.* Dobbs Ferry, NY: Morgan and Morgan, Inc; 1965.

Enkerud D. Understanding accommodative response. *J Biol Photog.* 1989;57:53-55.

Gass DJ. *Stereoscopic Atlas of Macular Disease.* St. Louis, Mo: CV Mosby Co; 1987.

Gibson HL. *Medical Photography.* Rochester, NY: Eastman Kodak; 1973.

Horenstein H. *Beyond Basic Photography: A Technical Manual.* Boston, Mass: Little, Brown, and Co; 1977.

Horenstein H. *Black and White Photography: A Basic Manual.* Boston, Mass: Little, Brown, and Co; 1983.

Horenstein H. *Color Photography: A Working Manual.* Boston, Mass: Little, Brown, and Co; 1995.

Justice J, ed. *Ophthalmic Photography.* Boston, Mass: Little, Brown, and Co; 1982.

Kogelman S and Heller BR. *The Only Math Book You'll Ever Need.* New York, NY: Facts on File Publications; 1986.

Mayer DJ. *Clinical Wide-field Specular Microscopy.* London: Bailliere Tindall; 1984.

Merin LM. The ophthalmic darkroom. In: Saine PJ, Tyler ME. *Ophthalmic Photography: A Textbook of Retinal Photography, Angiography, and Electronic Imaging.* Boston, Mass: Butterworth-Heinemann; 1997:169-199.

Merin L. Photography request forms. Journal of *Ophthalmic Photography.* 1984;7:88-92.

Morris PF. Fluorescein sodium and indocyanine green: uses and side effects. In: Saine PJ, Tyler ME. *Ophthalmic Photography: A Textbook of Retinal Photography, Angiography, and Electronic Imaging.* Boston, Mass: Butterworth-Heinemann; 1997:117-121.

Provenzo EF Jr, Provenzo AB. *Rediscovering Photography.* La Jolla, Calif: Oak Tree Publications, Inc; 1980.

Richards EP, Rathbun KC. *Law and the Physician: A Practical Guide.* Boston, Mass: Little, Brown and Co; 1993.

Robl EH. *Organizing Your Photographs.* New York, NY: Amphoto; 1986.

Rubin ML. *Optics for Clinicians.* Gainesville, Fla: Triad Scientific Publishers; 1977.

Ryan SJ. *Retina.* St. Louis, Mo: CV Mosby Co; 1994.

Saine PJ, Tyler ME. *Ophthalmic Photography: A Textbook of Retinal Photography, Angiography, and Electronic Imaging.* Boston, Mass: Butterworth-Heinemann; 1997.

Schatz H, Burton TC, Yannuzzi LA, Rabb MF. *Interpretation of Fundus Fluorescein Angiography.* St. Louis, Mo: CV Mosby Co; 1978.

Schatz H. *Essential Fluorescein Angiography.* Anselmo, Calif: Pacific Medical Press; 1983.

Shipman C. *Understanding Photography*. Tucson, Ariz: HP Books; 1974.

Stroebel L, Compton J, Current I, Zakia R. *Photographic Materials and Processes*. Boston, Mass: Focal Press; 1986.

Strohlein A. *The Management of 35 mm Medical Slides*. New York, NY: United Business Publications; 1975.

Vestal D. *The Craft of Photography*. New York, NY: Harper & Row Publishers; 1975.

Vetter JP, ed. *Biomedical Photography*. Boston, Mass; Butterworth-Heinemann; 1992.

Williams R. *Medical Photography Study Guide*. Hingham, Mass: MTP Press; 1984.

Wong D. The Fundus Camera. In: Tasman W, ed. *Duane's Clinical Ophthalmology*. Philadelphia, Pa: JB Lippincott Co; 1994:1-14.

Wong D. *Textbook of Ophthalmic Photography*. Birmingham, Ala: Inter-Optics Publications, Inc; 1982.

Yannuzzi LA, Rohrer KT, Tindel LJ, et al. Fluorescein angiography complication survey. *Ophthalmology*. 1986;3:611-617.

Index

For your information

This book and many others on numerous different topics are available from SLACK Incorporated. For further information or a copy of our latest catalog, contact us at:

Professional Book Division
SLACK Incorporated
6900 Grove Road
Thorofare, NJ 08086 USA
Telephone: 1-609-848-1000
1-800-257-8290
Fax: 1-609-853-5991
E-mail: orders@slackinc.com
WWW: http://www.slackinc.com

We accept most major credit cards and checks or money orders in US dollars drawn on a US bank. Most orders are shipped within 72 hours.

Contact us for information on recent releases, forthcoming titles, and bestsellers. If you have a comment about this title or see a need for a new book, direct your correspondence to the Editorial Director at the above address.

If you are an instructor, we can be reached at the address listed above or on the Internet at **educomps@slackinc.com** for specific needs.

Thank you for your interest and we hope you found this work beneficial.